D1612718

Charnley Low-Frictional Torque Arthroplasty of the Hip

B.M. Wroblewski • Paul D. Siney
Patricia A. Fleming

Charnley Low-Frictional Torque Arthroplasty of the Hip

Practice and Results

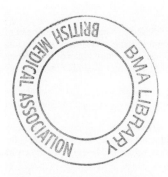

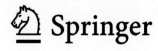

B.M. Wroblewski
The John Charnley Research Institute
Wrightington Hospital
Wigan, Lancashire
UK

Patricia A. Fleming
The John Charnley Research Institute
Wrightington Hosptial
Wigan, Lancashire
UK

Paul D. Siney
The John Charnley Research Institute
Wrightington Hospital
Wigan, Lancashire
UK

ISBN 978-3-319-21319-4   ISBN 978-3-319-21320-0   (eBook)
DOI 10.1007/978-3-319-21320-0

Library of Congress Control Number: 2016934314

Springer Cham Heidelberg New York Dordrecht London

Printed on acid-free paper

Springer International Publishing AG Switzerland is part of Springer Science+Business Media
(www.springer.com)

Foreword by Lady Charnley

At the time of Sir John's death in 1982, the Charnley low-friction arthroplasty for hip replacement was accepted as a great breakthrough and successful operation for patients suffering from arthritic hips. The procedure was not without its critics and the team, under the leadership of Professor Wroblewski, have carefully evaluated the results and problems over the years. They are to be congratulated for producing a book which will be invaluable to orthopaedic surgeons who seek to understand the underlying philosophy of the Charnley LFA.

Lady Charnley
President
The John Charnley Trust
McMillan & Co LLP
Chorley, Lancashire
UK

Foreword by Charnley Research Institute

Fifteen of the Fellows were from the UK and Ireland, John Hodgkinson, David Allen, David Beverland, Anthony Browne, Martin Stone, Shiv Gupta, Peter Kay, Videsh Raut, Mike Manning, Anthony Clayson, Eric Gardner, Roger Tillman, Chris Walker, Keith Barnes and Andrew Phillipson.

Four Fellows were from Europe, Blaise Wyssa, Rabih Makarem, Peter Bobak and Bodo Purbach.

Two Fellows were from North and South America, Alberto Dominguez and Major Greg Taylor.

Three Fellows were from Australia, Julian Lane, Scott Crawford and David Mitchell.

The last Fellow Hagime Nagai from Japan completed his fellowship in 2002.

Scott Crawford and Hajime Nagai had followed their respective fathers, Bill Crawford and Jun Nagai, who had both worked with Charnley at Wrightington in the 1960s.

Foreword

John Charnley's scientific development of the modern, successful, total hip arthroplasty must be considered one of medicine's greatest achievements in the twentieth century. His low-frictional torque arthroplasty has demonstrated enduring success since 1962 and established a turning point in orthopaedic surgery, from fractures and deformity to a discipline that offers some of the technically most challenging operations on almost all joints.

The operation has helped many thousands of patients all over the world to carry on with life in a way that was previously unthinkable. It was Charnley's well-calculated expectation that the replacement of the human hip joint could last up to 25 years. Today, it is possible to study the effect of joint replacements on the human skeleton up to 50 years. It has always been Charnley's understanding that the artificial replacement would fail eventually either because of wear in the bearing or failure of fixation within the skeleton. These changes can be anticipated but need to be monitored by long-term review.

The evaluation of long-term success – and failure – goes beyond a single surgeons' working-life experience, and it now befalls on the third generation of surgeons after Charnley to learn from the knowledge gathered over the last 50 years. Charnley established an apprenticeship-like teaching method, allowing surgeons worldwide to visit Wrightington and then disseminate the highly successful operation worldwide. The principles of Charnley's operation remain crucial to its long-term success, an approach to the hip using a trochanteric osteotomy, fixation and uniform load transfer using bone cement and a hard on soft small bearing to reduce the frictional torque on the fixation within the skeleton. The improvement of the operation has been the purpose and achievement of Professor Mike Wroblewski, the surgeon to continue with the evolution of Charnley's operation, principles and philosophy. It is the culmination of these achievements that is presented here, not as a success story that praises the results of the past but in the spirit of Professor Sir John Charnley, to foster a modern understanding of successful and failing designs of the artificial hip.

From the experience at Wrightington, the success of the hip replacement does not primarily rely on materials, but on the principles of the operation and the skill and technique of the surgeon.

This instructive and precise manual will most likely endure, if the bias in trends of modern and fashionable orthopaedics is replaced with a wish for a better understanding of success for the next generation of surgeons.

Bodo Purbach MD
Consultant Orthopaedic Surgeon
Centre for Hip Surgery
Wrightington Hospital
UK

Preface

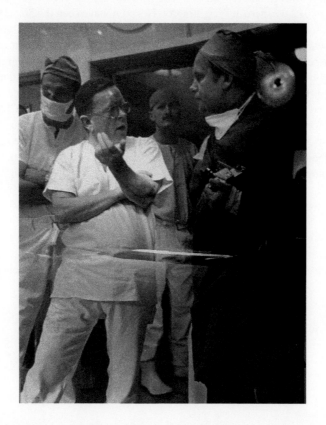

Photograph taken in 1970 of Professor Sir John Charnley in discussion with visiting surgeons in the operating theatre at Wrightington Hospital.

The purpose of this work is to offer a better understanding of the Charnley low-frictional torque arthroplasty of the hip: based on over 50 years of clinical experience.

The underlying principles and their practical application, evolution in the light of clinical experience, radiographic appearances and the examination of explanted components are all an integral part of that process. Changes in the design, surgical technique and even the materials were dictated by the detailed study of all aspects of the procedure and follow-up. Radical departures from the principles were never part of that process. We have remained faithful to the concept of low-frictional torque – the small diameter (22.225 mm) head of the femoral component articulating with a thick ultrahigh molecular weight polyethylene (UHMWPE) cup, both components grouted with cold curing acrylic cement polymethyl methacrylate (PMMA).

Exposure of the hip by trochanteric osteotomy has remained the method of choice.

Charnley, unfortunately, did not live to see the 20-year clinical results. In November 2012 we, here at Wrightington Hospital, have seen the 50-year milestone of the clinical application of the Charnley method. With the availability of long-term successes, and failures, it was, and still is, possible to focus attention on the various aspects of the operation, identify the problems and introduce changes accordingly. It is through the knowledge of the past and the understanding of the present that we can aim to achieve even better results for the future.

We hope that this record of the continuing evolution of the Charnley low-frictional torque arthroplasty (LFTA) – (more commonly known as low-friction arthroplasty, LFA) – will help the newcomer to the speciality to appreciate the reasons for the success of the operation, while the experienced members will use it a stepping stone for further improvement without the trauma of past experiences.

Wrightington, Lancashire, UK   B.M. Wroblewski

Wrightington, Lancashire, UK   Paul D. Siney

Wrightington, Lancashire, UK   Patricia A. Fleming

"The challenge comes when patients between 45 and 50 years of age are considered for the operation because then every advance in the technical details must be used if there is to be a reasonable chance of 20 or more years of trouble free activity".
"It is not in a young patient's interest for a surgeon to count on a successful 'revision' should mechanical failure ensue earlier than was expected".

Charnley 1979

Acknowledgements

When attempting to express thanks, any author faces a dilemma of "attempting to name them all" and the "fear of omitting some". No such problems here.

The late Mr Peter Kershaw of the Peter Kershaw Trust made the concept of the John Charnley Research Institute a reality. It continues to function and expand thanks to the unfailing support of the Trust. To Lady Charnley, who through the John Charnley Trust gave practical and moral support. To the fellows who became involved in this work, often at an inconvenience to their families.

To Mr Frank Brown, who worked in the Bio-Mechanical Laboratory for 40 years and with his practical knowledge of engineering and tool-making made instruments, modified implants and made prototypes, often from a rough sketch or even a discussion, as drawings, in the strict sense of the word, were never made.

To my secretary Brenda Lowerson, who after many years of hard work continued well beyond her duty often to the exclusion of her favourite golf.

Individuals who made specific contributions are acknowledged in the appropriate chapters.

To members of our families for their patience, understanding and support.

To patients who continue to be the integral part of the long-term follow-up studies. It is their commitment that paved the way to advancement of the Charnley low-frictional torque arthroplasty.

The John Charnley Research Institute Registered Charity 1099185.

Contents

Part I
Evolution of the Charnley Low Frictional Torque Arthroplasty

Chapter 1
The Concept of Total Hip Arthroplasty: The Beginning

"The only operation that ever could be universal would be an arthroplasty, because this is a reconstruction of a normal joint" 1959

Charnley's interest in the mechanics of the hip joint started early – whilst still a medical student. Later Charnley wrote *"the hip joint, which is an almost perfect ball and socket, is frequently affected by types of arthritis which destroy the rubbing surfaces and distort the geometry of the concentric spherical surfaces, with the result that motion is restricted and pain develops."*

Past attempts to replace one or both surfaces offered only a short term solution; *"...failure can be most commonly traced to the failure to maintain a sound mechanical bond between the artificial part (the prosthesis) ... and the living bone."*

Charnley identified the problems of arthritis as: failure of geometry commonly referred to as "worn joint" clinically presenting as pain, restriction of movement of the joint and patient's mobility.

Synovial fluid lubrication of normal joints was the accepted theory. The only published experimental work on lubrication of animal joints was that of Dr E Shirley Jones (Fig. 1.1) – (Joint Lubrication: *Lancet* 1936: 1; 1043).

Charnley corresponded with Dr Jones (Fig. 1.2) on the subject. It may, therefore, be of some interest to refer to some of the experimental work by Dr Jones (Figs. 1.3, 1.4, 1.5, and 1.6) on the subject.

The detailed analysis and the interpretation of the experimental work, both that of Jones and Charnley is outside the scope of this work; our interest lies in the evolution of the concept of the Charnley hip replacement.

© Springer International Publishing Switzerland 2016
B.M. Wroblewski et al., *Charnley Low-Frictional Torque Arthroplasty of the Hip: Practice and Results*, DOI 10.1007/978-3-319-21320-0_1

Fig. 1.1 Photograph of
Dr E.S. Jones

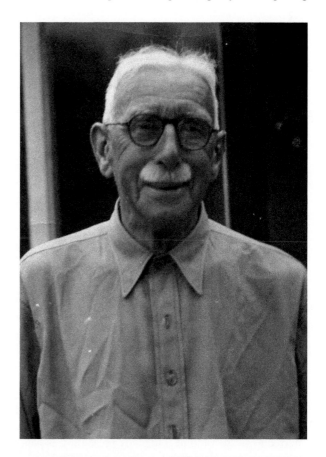

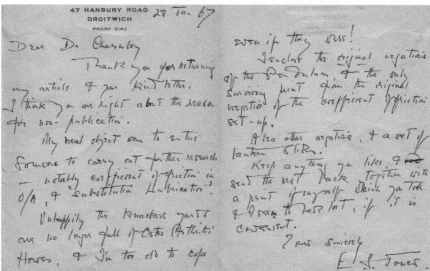

Fig. 1.2 Letter to Charnley from Dr ES Jones

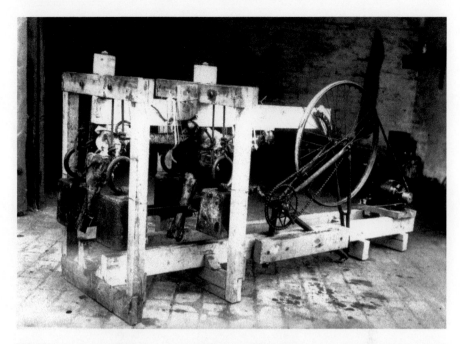

Fig. 1.3 Jones' experimental work on measuring coefficient of friction and lubrication in animal joints

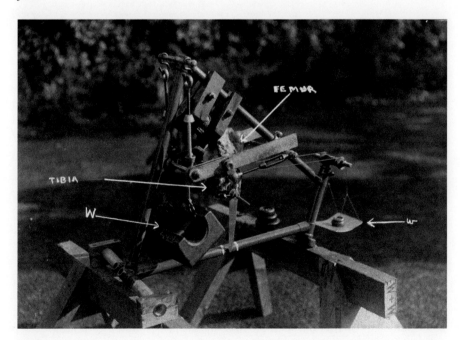

Fig. 1.4 Jones' experimental work on measuring coefficient of friction and lubrication in animal joints

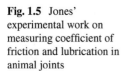

Fig. 1.5 Jones'
experimental work on
measuring coefficient of
friction and lubrication in
animal joints

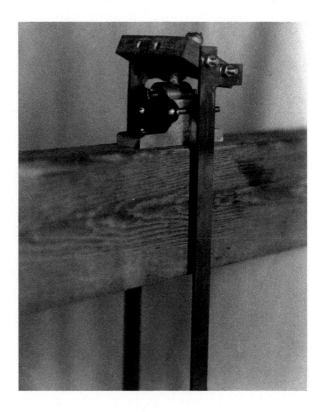

Lubrication

Charnley offered evidence for various possible modes of joint lubrication and suggested that if fluid film lubrication was the method that prevailed, then materials used for the replacement of joint surfaces would be less important than the geometry and viscosity of the lubricating fluid. He was in favour of hydrodynamic lubrication of natural joints; "*… a lubricant has an affinity for the surface it lubricates so that when motion takes place between two such lubricated surfaces it takes place between mono-molecular films of lubricant chemically adherent to the underlying surface*" (1959).

The likely mechanism by which metal on metal articulation may be lubricated "*… is explained by soaps being formed between the fatty acids and the metal with the result that the motion takes place between the two layers of molecules their COOH groups attached to the metal surface and the fatty chain projecting like the bristles of a brush*" (1959).

Charnley concluded that "*attempts to lubricate any artificial joint must be based on using boundary lubrication*"

Charnley attempted to simulate nature and followed the long accepted facts: low coefficient of friction: as a possible mechanical solution to a arthritic hip joint. "*I have collected the evidence to show that the coefficient of friction of normal articulate cartilage is phenomenally low and in fact lower than anything encountered between solid substances in engineering practice … The idea behind*

Fig. 1.6 Jones'
experimental work on
measuring coefficient of
friction and lubrication in
animal joints

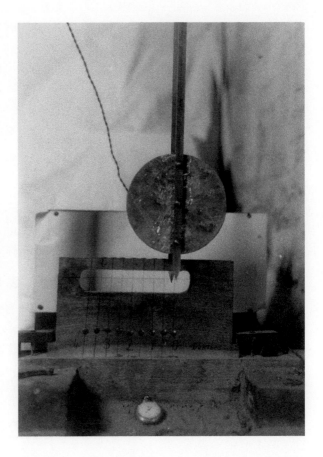

*the use of a low friction substance in arthroplasty is not merely in an endeavour
to eliminate wear on the surface of the prosthesis … the low friction concept
would eliminate any twisting stresses being transmitted to the bond between the
prosthesis and the living bone as a result of frictional resistance in the hip when
walking"* (1959). This reasoning was further supported by, and even possibly an
impetus for, the clinical application – in the form of the earliest attempt at hip
arthroplasty.

*"The starting point of the present research was the well known observation that
after the Judet operation the hip sometimes squeaks* (Figs. 1.7 and 1.8) *A squeak
indicated that frictional resistance to sliding is so high that the surfaces are seizing
together … investigations indicated that to give an artificial joint the same kind of
slipperiness as a natural joint, we should need a substance with a low coefficient of
friction which at the same time could well be tolerated by body tissues. For this
purpose I chose polytetrafluoroethylene (PTFE), a plastic which looks not unlike
cartilage and is chemically the most inert plastic so far discovered"* (1960). *"… in
my initial experiments with PTFE I used this substance as a synthetic cartilage …
It was hoped that motion would take place preferentially between two slippery
PTFE surfaces rather than between one PTFE surface and the bone …"*

Fig. 1.7 Radiograph of a
Judet prosthesis

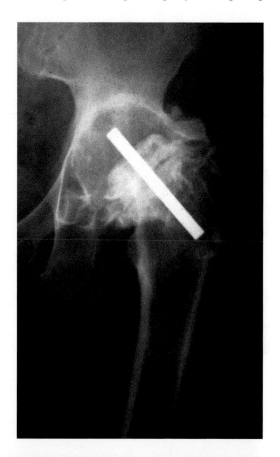

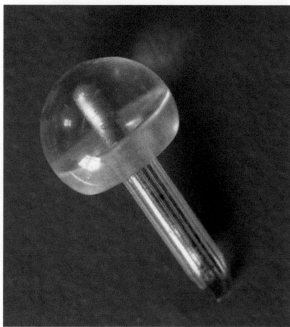

Fig. 1.8 Photograph of a
Judet prosthesis

This was the first attempt at double shell resurfacing arthroplasty. The acetabulum and the head of the femur were shaped with purpose designed instruments. The spigot of the acetabular reamer served first for centering then for locating the acetabular PTFE shell. The femoral head was likewise capped with a PTFE cup (Fig. 1.9). Charnley hoped that *"the movement will take place primarily between the PTFE articulating surfaces while, with time, bone will grow into the grooves fashioned for the purpose"*. Although Charnley refers to this period of his work as *"… my initial experiments"* these were clearly clinical experiments: patients undergoing operative procedures of PTFE double shell resurfacing arthroplasty.

And yet, it must not be concluded that Charnley did not give much thought to the subject of tissue reaction to new materials. *"I have introduced subcutaneously into my thigh, by means of a wide bore needle …two specimens of PTFE prepared in finely divided form. After nine months … the two specimens are clearly palpable and have been stationary in size for the last six months"* [1]. Histology slides of the excised implant clearly document the facts (Figs. 1.10 and 1.11).

What conclusions were or could have been drawn from these early experiments? The one that must be now obvious to all was that PTFE resurfacing shell arthroplasty, not only wore very rapidly at both interfaces, but also resulted in extensive bone destruction. The less obvious one and certainly of greater value as to future developments was the clinical success. Freedom from pain was remarkable even if

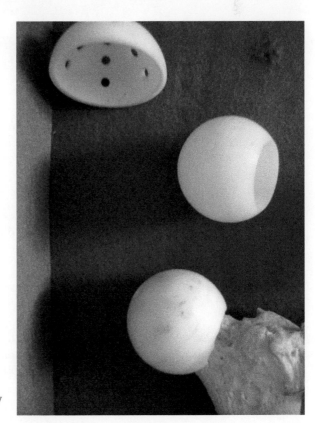

Fig. 1.9 Charnley's double shell resurfacing arthroplasty using PTFE

Fig. 1.10 Histology taken
from PTFE specimens
from Charnley's thigh

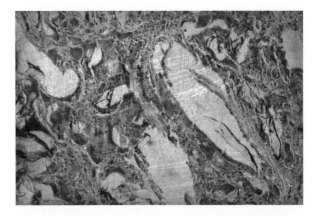

Fig. 1.11 Histology taken
from PTFE specimens
from Charnley's thigh

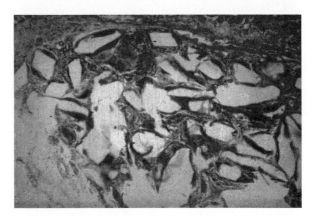

only short lasting. *"Very good immediate post-operative result lasted about six months"* (entry in Hip Register 11/02/1960). The first demanded closer attention to the plastic – PTFE – the second was a spur to persevere with the efforts of hip replacement.

From Double Shell Resurfacing to Cemented Stem and PTFE Cup

> *"It is probable that in future developments, prosthetic replacement of the femoral head, articulating with a PTFE cup, will prove more desirable than the double concentric shells of PTFE"* (1960)

Charnley was already familiar with the treatment of fractures of the neck of the femur using cemented Moore and Thompson hemi-arthroplasty. It is, therefore, logical that this aspect, the cemented femoral head replacement, be incorporated into the next stage.

Fig. 1.12 Subcutaneous injections of Chrome, Nickel and Cobalt (June–July 1974)

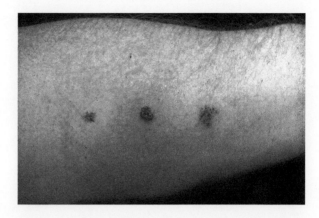

"… *I had used a standard Moore prosthesis with a ball of 1⁵/₈ in diameter believing that PTFE being a relatively soft material would wear longer if the load per unit area of the bearing surface were the smallest possible…*". Charnley again experimented on himself (Fig. 1.12).

The stages in the evolution of the operation were documented in the *Lancet.* [2].

"*Between 1958 and 1960 the maximum diameter ball which anatomical considerations would permit (41.5 mm) was chosen to replace the femoral head. This left only 5 mm as the maximum wall thickness of the plastic cup.*" Early clinical success was followed by problems; "*discomfort returned*". Exploring the failed hips Charnley found that "*the PTFE socket tended to move with the large steel ball … the phenomenal slipperiness attributed to PTFE in the laboratory appeared not to hold after some months in the human body …the most serious aspect of the failure of the PTFE was the tissue reaction to wear debris.*" This was really not so much "*tissue reaction to wear debris*" but the result of PTFE wear directly on bone.

References

1. Waugh W. In: John Charnley, editor. The man and the hip. London: Springer; 1990. p. 121.
2. Charnley J. Arthroplasty of the hip. A new operation. Lancet. 1961 (May 27):1129–32.

Chapter 2
Arthroplasty of the Hip: A New Operation

From Low Friction to Low Frictional Torque

"In a design of a load bearing joint I have rather lost interest in the coefficient of friction between the materials of the rubbing surfaces as a guiding factor in design. It is possible to circumvent the coefficient of friction by concentrating on low-frictional torque in the assembled unit by reducing the diameter of the ball" ... *"It was pointed out to me that the best engineering practice would be to use the smallest diameter ball which could cope with the expected load. Resistance to movement of the head in the socket is greatly reduced by reducing the radius of the ball and therefore reducing the "moment" of the frictional force. If, at the same time, the radius of the exterior of the PTFE socket is made as large as possible, the "moment" of the frictional force between the socket and the bone will be increased and this will lessen the tendency for the socket to rotate against bone. The result of reducing the size of the femoral head was to prolong the period during which the success was absolute."* ... *"Since there was no way of estimating rigours of service in the human hip joint over a period of years, we had to proceed by trial and error ... from the starting size of 41.5 mm diameter ... this was first reduced to 28.5 mm then 25.25 mm and finally to 22 mm"* (actually 22.225 mm or 7/8 in.) (1966) (Fig. 2.1). Charnley worked with the then standard Imperial System. The first recorded LFA using $^7/_8$ in. (22.225 mm) head diameter in the Charnley Hip Register is dated 29.09.1960. *"Fluon socket arthroplasty – left hip – using $^7/_8$ in. prosthesis long neck.*

It is this change of concept from "low-friction" the property of the materials to "low-frictional torque" the principle of the design, that marks the fundamental turning point in the evolution of the low-frictional torque arthroplasty; henceforth referred to as the Charnley LFA (Fig. 2.2).

© Springer International Publishing Switzerland 2016
B.M. Wroblewski et al., *Charnley Low-Frictional Torque Arthroplasty of the Hip: Practice and Results*, DOI 10.1007/978-3-319-21320-0_2

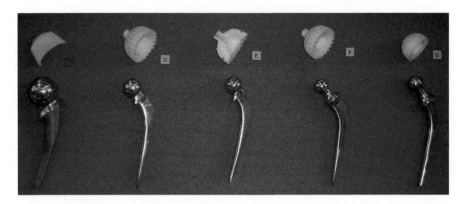

Fig. 2.1 Reducing the diameter of the head of the femoral component from 41.5 down to 22.225 mm

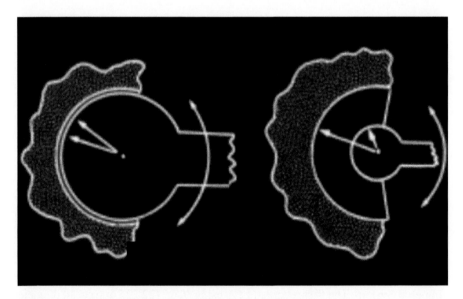

Fig. 2.2 Low frictional torque principle. Difference in the radii of small femoral head with socket of maximum external diameter

Charnley, however, continued using PTFE as the material for the cup. Charnley discussed *"low frictional arthroplasty"* and its application in rheumatoid arthritis, geriatrics and as a primary procedure in fractures of the neck of the femur. Detailing the operative technique Charnley states *"a low-friction socket in Teflon … cemented in position using cold-curing acrylic cement"*. (1965) [1].

The "Teflon Era"

Charnley's experience with Teflon is, unfortunately, better known for the failures than the contributions made to the development of hip replacement. It was during that period that the design of the components, *"the mechanical details of the technique became stabilised in the period 1959–1962 in the Teflon era ..."* (1971) wear characteristics and tissue reaction to PTFE wear particles, histology of bone-cement interface were established. Material suitable for the cup was the one missing link.

Kamangar et al. [2] studied 100 PTFE "pressfit" cups in an attempt to find information supporting the low-frictional torque principle. Majority of the cups, 72, were articulating with the 22.225 mm diameter head, 12 with 25.25 mm, 12 with 28.5 mm and 4 with 41.5 mm diameter heads. Of the 100 cups 58 were not completely worn through; 39 were articulating with 22.225 mm, 11 with 25.25 mm, 6 with 28.5 mm and 2 with 41.5 mm diameter heads. Charnley could not have hoped to find the information he was seeking: Long term successful results would not have been possible, all cups were taken from revisions, they were worn and loose, numbers were small and follow-up short to allow comparison of results with various head sizes. Yet, even when examining failures, Charnley did find very valuable information.

"The most serious aspect of the failure of PTFE was the production of tissue reaction by wear debris"

"wear of the PTFE socket seemed to be more dependent on the activity of the patient than the weight ..."

"... the wear of the plastic sockets took place by the steel ball boring into the substance of the plastic to make a cylindrical pathway of the same diameter as the steel head ..."

"the rate of volumetric wear found must be directly proportional to the diameter of the sphere..."

"It is concluded that, from consideration of the geometry and the wear characteristics of metal spheres in plastic sockets, the sphere should have a diameter not greater than half that of the external convex diameter of the socket." (1969); the fundamental basis of the Charnley concept.

The most important, and probably the least known observation, was that the operation was immediately successful – freedom from pain was complete. Patients were prepared to accept further surgery even if the freedom from pain was no more than several years.

The operation had to be abandoned because of rapid wear of the PTFE cups and gross destruction of bone. During this period of despondency cemented Thompson hemi-arthroplasty was used in some cases where the relatively well preserved acetabulum permitted. Such cases were relatively few.

It must be appreciated that by the time PTFE was abandoned the concept of the low-frictional torque arthroplasty was fully established. Not only that – the design and methods of manufacture of the components, including the lapping and polishing of the 22.225 mm diameter head in EN58J stainless steel, but also a full range of instruments and the details of surgical technique were in place. Documentation of clinical assessment, operative details and the study of results of this type of surgery and the Hip Register were also fully established. The one missing link was suitable material for the cup.

Statements, Comments and Lessons from the Past: Extracts from Charnley's Hip Register 1959–1961

31.03.60	Revision of double cup left hip arthroplasty. *"This confirms the impression that the second operation is, by and large, disappointing".*
29.09.60	*"Fluon socket arthroplasty left hip using ⁷/₈ in. prosthesis long neck".* (First recorded case using ⁷/₈ in. (22.225 mm) diameter stainless steel head).
15.06.61	Disarticulation left hip: *"This case demonstrates the disastrous effects of sepsis in implant prosthetic surgery."* (The only such case).
22.11.62	*Low friction arthroplasty Cup: NEW 1⁷/₈ in..* (First documented UHMWPE Cup).

Ultra High Molecular Weight Polyethylene as the Material for the Cup

"I was not interested and said so in no uncertain terms. But my technician (Harry Craven) *hating to see the apparatus idle, and unknown to me, loaded the apparatus with four specimens of the new material. After three weeks of day to day running, the test had not worn as much as we would have expected in one day using polytetrafluoroethylene. From that moment the game was on."*

"I am rather optimistic about the properties of the new plastic High Molecular Weight Polyethylene. The coefficient of friction is not particularly low but by mechanical design, the frictional resistance of the unit can be made very low." (Charnley recalling events in 1974) (Fig. 2.3)

Information gathered from various sources, including a representative of the distributor, would suggest that ultra high molecular weight polyethylene was introduced, into the UK from Germany, sometime in 1960. It was the result of a combination of factors: the protection of buffalo in the United States and the advent of man-made fibre. Buffalo hide was hitherto used in industry for the manufacture of conveyor belts and washers; the animal was now being protected. Fine, regular texture of man-made fibre was readily spoiled by inclusion of hide shards; High molecular weight polyethylene was the alternative and also very suitable for the manufacture of gears. Charnley *"… was assured by the manufacturers of RCH1000 that this product contains no more than 100 ppm of impurities comprising retained*

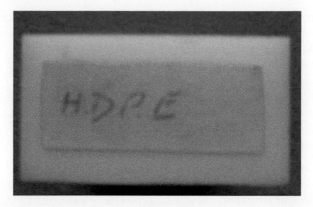

Fig. 2.3 Specimen of high density polyethylene from 1962

catalyst of metallic chlorides (aluminium, titanium, sodium and potassium). The anti-oxidant has not been divulged by the manufacturer." (1974) There is no record detailing the quality of UHMWPE as used in clinical practice from the time of its introduction in November 1962. The first HDP cup was implanted on 22/11/1962. What is documented is the source of the material: *"The high molecular weight poly-ethylene came from the same source as the early series."* (1978): there was continuity of the supplier and with it, presumably, of the manufacturing process and, therefore, consistency of the quality of the material.

During the period November 1962–March 1967, the cups were machined by Harry Craven in Charnley's workshop. The machined cups were washed, soaked in formaldehyde overnight, and washed again before implantation. Whether this process had any effect on the wear rate of the UHMWPE is not known. (In the 135 hips replaced between 1962 and 1965, the mean penetration rate was 0.15 mm/year at a follow-up of 9–10 years. Comparable results have been obtained in subsequent series).

From March 1967 the production of UHMWPE cups was taken over by Charles F Thackray, Leeds, U.K. and from then on the cups were sterilised by gamma irradiation, in air.

From 1998 UHMWPE cups had been gamma irradiated in nitrogen. If some confusion occurred in the early stage it is probably because the product material was labelled, for a short period of time, incorrectly, as PTFE although it was in fact RCH1000.

Acutely aware of problems with PTFE, Charnley continued detailed studies of UHMWPE wear. In the 1967–1968 series, 547 LFAs were included with a mean follow-up of 8.3 years (range 7–9 years) *"the average wear* (total penetration) *was 0.59 mm representing an annual average rate of 0.07 mm/year"* (1978).

The information obtained from the study led to the following conclusions:

Gender: *"males appear to be more likely to show greater wear than females"*

Age: *"...there were no significant differences in the age group of patients showing mild to intermediate wear...the incidence of heavy wear was more directly related to the age of the patients."*

Weight: *"There was ... no direct correlation between the weight of the patient and the amount of wear."*

Function: *"... there is evidence that physical activity in young male patients is associated with high wear rates ... it appears that unless the function is grade 6* (normal) *for several years heavy wear does not occur."* These findings confirmed the information previously gathered with PTFE.

Surface finish of the head of the femoral component: *"The arthroplasties ... performed in 1966 were excluded* (from the 1978 study) *because during 1966 the source of femoral prostheses has changed from those where the head had been finished in our experimental laboratories to those finished professionally."*

Sphericity and Surface Finish of the 22.225 mm Diameter Stainless Steel Head

There is documented evidence that both sphericity and surface finish of the metal head were of special interest to Charnley; comparisons with other designs were frequently made in the Biomechanical Laboratory at Wrightington Hospital. Once the manufacture was taken over by Charles F Thackray, Leeds, U.K. in 1967 it became their responsibility to comply with the set standards. It is not clear what, if any, standards were laid down at that stage. What is clear, however, that the British and International Standards, established later, were not only achieved but also maintained in clinical practice, when stems taken from revisions, were examined.

Compared with rapidly wearing PTFE, UHMWPE did not appear to pose any foreseeable problems, certainly not observed in the early results. There were other issues to be addressed – fractured stem presenting as a sudden failure. It was those cases that demanded immediate attention. Questions concerning materials, design and surgical technique of stem fixation had to be addressed urgently. With increasing follow-up it became clear that wear and loosening of the UHMWPE was the most likely long-term problem – as predicted by Charnley: ... *"The late failure, if it does eventually supervene, is to be expected from one, or both, of the two possible causes: Tissue reaction to particles abraded from the bearing surfaces; and mechanical loosening of the cement bond in the bone."* (1961).

Acrylic Cement

"The crux of this operation ... lies in the use of cement. By means of cement the load of the body weight is distributed over a large area of bone"

"Acrylic cement does not adhere to bone like glue it merely forms an accurate cast of the interior of the bone so that the load is transmitted evenly over all parts of the interface between cement and cancellous bone."

"I was not the first to use acrylic cement in attempting to bond orthopaedic implants to bone, but I was the first to use it successfully." (1963)

These statements summarize succinctly all the aspects of the technique of component fixation using acrylic cement. The challenge now was to translate the concept into practical solutions through the study of materials and designs, but above all, the surgical technique based on the initial premise.

Bone Cement

Bone cements are based on methylmethacrylate (MMA), an ester of methacrylic acid. The original work of Otto Rohm led to the development of MMA dentures. The first "clinical" application of polymethylmethacrylate (PMMA) was an attempt to close experimentally produced cranial defects in monkeys, followed by its use in humans.

Degussa and Kulzer (1943) quoted by Kuhn [3] established a protocol for the chemical production of PMMA. Kiaer [4] and Haboush [5] are reputed to have been the first to use acrylic cement for component fixation. In both these attempts the acrylic cement was confined to the cancellous bone of the proximal femur.

Tissue reaction to PMMA was studied by Henrichsen and colleagues [6] and Wiltse and colleagues [7].

The Femur

In the 3 years following the original report Charnley had inserted 455 prostheses using acrylic cement. Six necropsy specimens were available. The histological appearances on the femoral side were encouraging *"... no sclerosis of cancellous bone ... cancellous bone repaired ... normal appearance of the cellular content of narrow spaces ... no fibrosis."* (1964)

References

1. Charnley J. Low friction arthroplasty of the hip joint. Prog Clin Rheumatol. 1965;339–47.
2. Kamangar A, Charnley J, Longfield MD. The optimum size of prosthetic heads in relation to the wear of plastic sockets in total replacement of the hip. Med Biol Eng. 1969;7:31–9.
3. Kuhn K-D. Bone cements. Up to date comparisons of physical and chemical properties of commercial material. New York: Springer; 2000.

4. Kiaer S. Preliminary report on arthroplasty by use of acrylic head. Stockholm: Chinguiem Congres International de Chirurgie Orthopedique; 1951.
5. Haboush EJA. A new operation for arthroplasty of the hip based on biomechanics, photoelasticity, fast-setting dental acrylic, and other considerations. Bull Hosp NY. 1953;14:242.
6. Henrichsen E, Jansen K, Krogh-Poulson W. Experimental investigation of the tissue reaction to acrylic plastics. Acta Orthop Scand. 1953;22:141–6.
7. Wiltse LL, Hall RH, Stoneheim JC. Experimental studies regarding the possible use of self-curing acrylic cement in orthopaedic surgery. J Bone Joint Surg. 1967;39-B:961–72.

Chapter 3
A New Surgical Science

A new surgical science – total prosthetic joint replacement – has suddenly come into being. A heavy work load has suddenly been created in response to the availability of a successful new operation … orthopaedic departments planned for the future district general hospital will be unable to cope if they are to handle the routine orthopaedics for which they were designed.

When one tries to consider how highly specialised techniques can best be made available to a large number of patients … one has to face the fact that it is impossible, now or at any time in the future, and even in the most wealthy countries, to avoid some type of rationing. Rationing will have to be a product of educating surgeons in the methods of assessing the priority for surgery and self-discipline in patients fostered by education. (1970)

Caution

Charnley was fully aware of the implications of a successful hip replacement with the likely future demands and responsibilities. Once again the "Teflon Experience" was not without practical benefits.

- *I am making no attempt to encourage other surgeons to adopt this procedure for at least another three or four years or until an authoritative body such as the British Orthopaedic Association might request it … the designs have not been made available to manufacturers…*
- *This operation must be reserved …for very disabled patients and the warning that a second operation might be necessary after some years … should be given. (1963)*

The seriousness of the procedure, the need for regular follow-up and monitoring of outcome, as well as provision of revision facilities, are well documented.

- *An important aspect of the use of total prosthetic replacement is acceptance by the patient of a planned policy of "revision" with the establishment of a centre which holds itself permanently responsible for maintenance of this type of surgery* and
- *I regard it mandatory that any surgeon aiming to take up the "total prosthesis" should make available to the public a service which can cope with the maintenance operations* (1966)

© Springer International Publishing Switzerland 2016
B.M. Wroblewski et al., *Charnley Low-Frictional Torque Arthroplasty of the Hip: Practice and Results*, DOI 10.1007/978-3-319-21320-0_3

- *To countenance the insertion of total hip replacement into a patient of 25 years of age in 1971, without a service station planned and organised for 1996, is like selling motor cars without providing mechanics and workshops.* (1971)

Charnley's views are succinctly summarised in a statement:

- *We have continuously to ask ourselves what type of late failure we must be prepared for, and we must protect patients too ready to submit to this practice after seeing patients who have been dramatically "cured" by this method. The past history of the arthroplasty of the hip joint is no great credit to orthopaedic surgery.* (1967)

Training

- *I visualise the establishment of a limited number of specialist centres such as this at Wrightington to train the postgraduates in the technology, to take problem cases, to cope with secondary operations…*
- *It is essential that the technical skills acquired by members of the staff of a surgical centre should be handed on continuously so as to keep a body of men capable of handling the difficult secondary operations of the future." "… by encouraging professionalism, by narrowing fields of activity, the quality of service can be raised and the cost per item lowered, … surgical residents turn out first class surgery because they are supported by a professional team which is not subject to continuous change.*
- *Uniform criteria can be established in large centres … the most dangerous unit is a small unit looking for work.*
- *We are ready to make contact with non-conforming minds, since this helps us to see our established techniques through non committed eyes.*
- *There is no sign of any trend towards copying the pattern established at Wrightington.*
- *Perhaps I am blind to defects of supreme specialization which may be obvious to others … perhaps for others the pressure of day-to-day work is obscuring trends which will soon require decisive action.*

Cost Implications

The demand for this type of surgery and the cost implications to the National Health Service were anticipated. The price of components was kept deliberately low. *"The NHS has to bear the costs."*

Charnley took no royalties and any financial benefits were channelled into research. Neither the design nor the methods of manufacture of the prosthetic components or the instruments were patented. It was the rapidly increasing demand and commercial pressure on the manufacturer in the face of mounting competition and copying that forced Charnley to allow the release of the LFA components, but not until the second half of 1970. Charnley informed the past Residents of his decision by a personal letter.

Statements made by Charnley many years ago serve as reminder of how far sighted he was.

Long-Term Follow-Up: The "First 500"

It was therefore decided upon to make a prospective study of those patients operated on between November 1962 and the end of December 1965 and to continue this annually until they could no longer attend. This would produce truly long-term studies ... (1970)

This attempt at *"truly long-term studies"* must be seen in the light of the continuing developments based on the ongoing clinical experience. All the operations carried out in the 3 year period November 1962 and December 1965, were included.

Some detailing of the various procedures is essential in order to offer a better understanding of the first 3 years in the history of the Charnley LFA.

Although referred to as the "FIRST 500" the total number of operations, and thus hips included, was 909. Patients' mean age at the operation was 65 years (range 22–86). The details are shown in Tables 3.1, 3.2, and 3.3.

Primary LFA There were 420 such procedures. Both the cup and the stem were fixed with acrylic cement. It is this group of 420 that was used as a "baseline" in subsequent studies.

Table 3.1 The Original "First 500" group selected by Charnley for an indefinite follow-up. All patients operated upon from November 1962 to December 1965 were included: 420 were primary LFAs

	LFA[a]	Press-fit cup[b]	Teflon to Press-fit	Teflon to LFA	Total
1962/1963	185	37	4	50	276
1964	47	193	18	40	298
1965	188	106		41	335
Total	420	336	22	131	909

[a]LFA: = cemented cup and stem
[b]Press-fit cup: = metal-backed cup with cemented stem

Table 3.2 "First 500" Press-fit cup group reviewed in 1983. Only 16 hips were available for follow-up

	Number	Died	Lost	Revised	Attending
1962/1963	37	21	10	4	2
1964	193	73	74	37	9
1965	106	30	44	27	5
Total	336	124	128	68	16
%	(100 %)	(36.9 %)	(38.1 %)	(20.2 %)	(4.8 %)

Table 3.3 "First 500" LFA group reviewed in 1983. Only 32 hips were available for follow-up

	Number	Died	Lost	Revised	Attending
1962/1963	185	88	66	13	18
1964	47	24	19	3	1
1965	188	78	86	11	13
Total	420	190	171	27	32
%	(100 %)	(45.2 %)	(40.7 %)	(6.4 %)	(7.6 %)

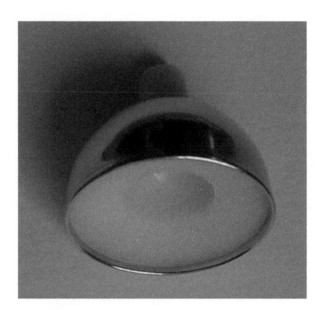

Fig. 3.1 Press-fit cup used without cement

Press-fit cup with cemented stem The design utilised the Smith-Peterson cup with an ultra high molecular weight polyethylene insert. An opening at the summit of the metal shell was machined into which a spigot of the UHMWPE cup would fit – protruding and thus serving as a locating guide into the pilot hole which was made in the acetabular floor as part of the reaming technique (Fig. 3.1).

The press-fit cup, not cemented in the acetabulum, though rigidly hammered into position at the time of the operation, the socket could rotate on its axis.

The reason for introducing the press-fit cup was "*the recognition by mid 1963 … that the demarcation between radio-opaque cement and the bone of the acetabulum was becoming a common radiological occurrence.*" The fear of the consequences of early demarcation of the bone-cement interface of the cup is reflected in the change of practice: out of 298 operations carried out in 1964, the press-fit cup was used in 211 (71 %). The press-fit cup was not used after 1965. From then on all cups were cemented because; "*demarcation of the cemented socket did not seem to be progressing beyond the amount visible at the end of the first year and ... ... a rather high rate of tilting and migration of the press-fit cup often leading to dislocation."* (It may be of interest to point out that one of the longest follow-up successful LFA's was in fact a patient with bilateral press-fit cups with cemented stem – past 40 years) (Figs. 3.2, 3.3 and 3.4).

In this group of "First 500" – there were 153 revisions: Teflon to press-fit – 22, Teflon to LFA – 131. Thus, out of a total of 909 operations, less than half: 420, (46 %), were primary LFAs in the true sense. By October 1977 *"over 100 of this original group were able to attend or keep in communication by questionnaire ... or by returning an annual radiograph taken near where they live."* (1979)

By 1983 only 48 hips: 32 LFAs and 16 with press-fit cups were available for follow-up. The dwindling numbers could provide only limited information that was essential to establish the clinical value of the operation but could not *"produce truly long-term studies"* as envisaged by Charnley.

It became clear that a new group of younger patients had to be selected. This decision was taken in 1974. **"Since 1974 we have had a policy that all patients aged 50 years or less at the time of the LFA are followed up indefinitely. Our reasons are life expectancy, the possibility of studying long-term outcomes, and the need for early intervention for impending failure"** [1]. Long-term follow-up can only be achieved with young patients.

Such a decision brings with it aspects hitherto not considered: changes in the patterns of underlying hip pathology, longer life expectations and higher activity level, more frequent follow-up and intervention for failures, both radiographic and clinical. And yet such a policy had to be put into practice, not only to establish the true long-term clinical value of the Charnley hip replacement, but also to investigate the patterns of problems to come and use them as pointers for new developments.

Clinical success of total hip arthroplasty is often taken for granted subject to correct patient selection and sound fixation of the components. Various methods of assessing the early clinical outcome serve as a reassurance of adequate patient selection for the operation by the surgeon and not a measure of long-term success of the method. Clinical results do not reflect the mechanical state of the arthroplasty: at this stage of our knowledge good quality radiographs are more valuable.

One other factor was to become very prominent with time – the cost of the follow-up. Yet how was the progress to be assessed? Charnley wrote in 1971 *"To countenance the insertion of total hip replacement into a patient of 25 years of age in 1971, without a service station organised for 1996, is like selling motor cars without providing mechanics and a workshop."* Should *"selling motor cars"* continue *"without providing mechanics and a workshop"* – the after sales service?

This volume is the confirmation of the Charnley principles; the continuing follow-up of patients under the age of 51 years; the operations carried out between November 1962 and December 1990.

The collection and study of information is a continuing process. Clinical results and radiographic appearances are updated at each follow-up. Findings at revisions

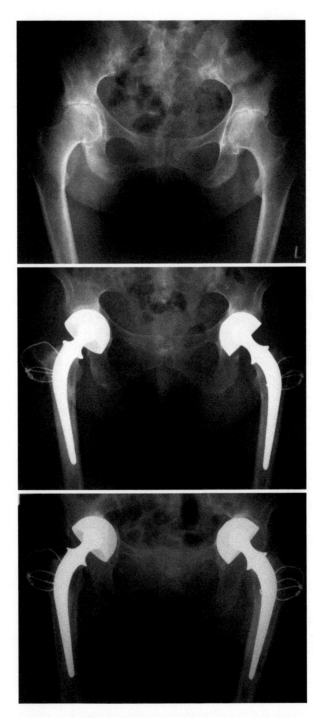

Figs. 3.2, 3.3 and 3.4 Radiographs of bilateral press-fit Cups. Pre-operative, post operative, and at 42 years after surgery

are recorded. Explanted components and soft tissues are studied in collaboration with Universities. Information gathered serves for the introduction of evidence-based improvements in design, materials and surgical techniques. Each aspect now becomes a study in its own right as patients are continually added to the inevitably dwindling original group.

Bone Cement Interphase Study. Examination of Post-Mortem Specimens

If we are to contemplate total hip replacement in adults as young as 45 years of age with the idea of 25 years of a trouble-free life ahead, it is necessary to hold definite opinions on the histological nature of the bone cement interface.

*At Wrightington Hospital by about 1965 it became obvious that it was imperative as soon as possible to obtain post-mortem material from **highly successful cases** ...*

The use of cement for component fixation and the study of the bone-cement interface has been an integral part of the concept, development and the technique of the Charnley LFA.

Charnley first used acrylic cement in 1958 for the fixation of femoral hemi-arthroplasties. Thirty five such procedures were carried out in the first year. *"The results were superior to those without cement"* [2].

Charnley considered that a lasting bond between bone and the acrylic cement could be achieved, certainly on the femoral if not acetabular side [3].

Aware of the clinical importance of long term histological studies Charnley approached a number of his patients with a very tactfully written request that their hip be bequeathed for post-mortem histological studies. Charnley prepared a letter explaining not only the need for the study but also accepting his own mortality (Figs. 3.5, 3.6 and 3.7). *"I would come by car with the necessary equipment to remove the specimen at the undertaker's premises..."*

Collection of Post Mortem Specimens

A standard metal box routinely used for sterilisation of various materials and instruments were ready for when a call came (Fig. 3.8). Either Charnley himself or the next available Senior Resident performed the duty.

Lateral incision down to the shaft of the femur, division of the femur – about mid-shaft – with the Gigli saw, then distal to proximal dissection of the femur, section of the pubic rami medially and the ilium posteriorly, skin closure. (The arthroplasty was not opened). The specimen thus secured was placed in the receptacle and filled with aqueous solution of formaldehyde on return to the Hip Centre.

TELEPHONE—APPLEY BRIDGE 521

WRIGHTINGTON HOSPITAL MANAGEMENT COMMITTEE
CENTRE FOR HIP SURGERY
WRIGHTINGTON HOSPITAL
Near WIGAN

1st August, 1966.

Dear

Private and Confidential

I am writing to some of my patients who have had the new operation, "low friction arthroplasty", performed on their hip, at least one year ago, to see whether they might be prepared to help me in medical research on this important problem of arthritis of the hip.

I am selecting patients whose ages are such that they are likely to predecease me by more than ten years, in the hope that they will bequeath their operated hip to medical research.

The great advances that we have made at Wrightington in the surgery of the hip joint are now established in the case of elderly patients, because elderly patients do not expose the artificial hip to the very great mechanical stresses which the hip experiences in middle and early middle age. One of the great problems we are faced with is the young woman (30 to 40 years of age), who has both hips stiff and painful as a result of being born with defective hip joints (congenital dislocation of the hips). Hips of this kind can survive the first 25 or 30 years of life without giving much trouble and then suddenly fail. We have no way of finding out if this new operation can be developed to suit this important group of patients unless we can get opportunities to study the sites where incipient defects are likely to develop after the artificial hip joint has been in position for a considerably number of years.

Animal experimentation in this work is of no use, because man is the only creature which walks with full weight on two legs. Experiments in the engineering laboratory in the same way are of restricted value because the most likely site of failure is likely to lie between the artificial hip and the living bone. It is quite easy to solve the mechanical problem inside the artificial hip joint itself in the engineering laboratory and we believe we have done this.

If the idea of making such a bequest should be repugnant to you, I sincerely hope you will forget this letter. In the case of your failure to reply to this letter I shall take precautions, through our records system, to make sure that you are never bothered again on this score.

If the idea of making this bequest appeals to you, (and I may say that it would be a noble gesture and of more value to research on the problems of younger patients than a donation of £250,000), the procedure to be adopted is quite simple and is as follows:-

1.   Sign where indicated at the bottom of this letter and retain this letter in your personal documents.

2.   Sign the copy of this letter which is enclosed, and return this copy in the stamped addressed envelope.

3.   Insert the name and address of your eldest son or daughter where indicated.

I have taken the decision to approach you directly on this topic because close relatives are always more disturbed about making a decision in this matter than are the patients themselves; indeed my attempts in the past to approach relatives on this matter so far have had only one successful outcome. I think that if it were known that a bequest of this kind was the earnest wish of their parent everyone would be happy to carry it out.

Kind regards,

Yours sincerely,

John Charnley, D.Sc., F.R.C.S.,
Consultant Orthopaedic Surgeon and
Director of Hip Surgery.

Fig. 3.5 Letter of bequeath from Charnley to his patients asking for their hip replacement after death

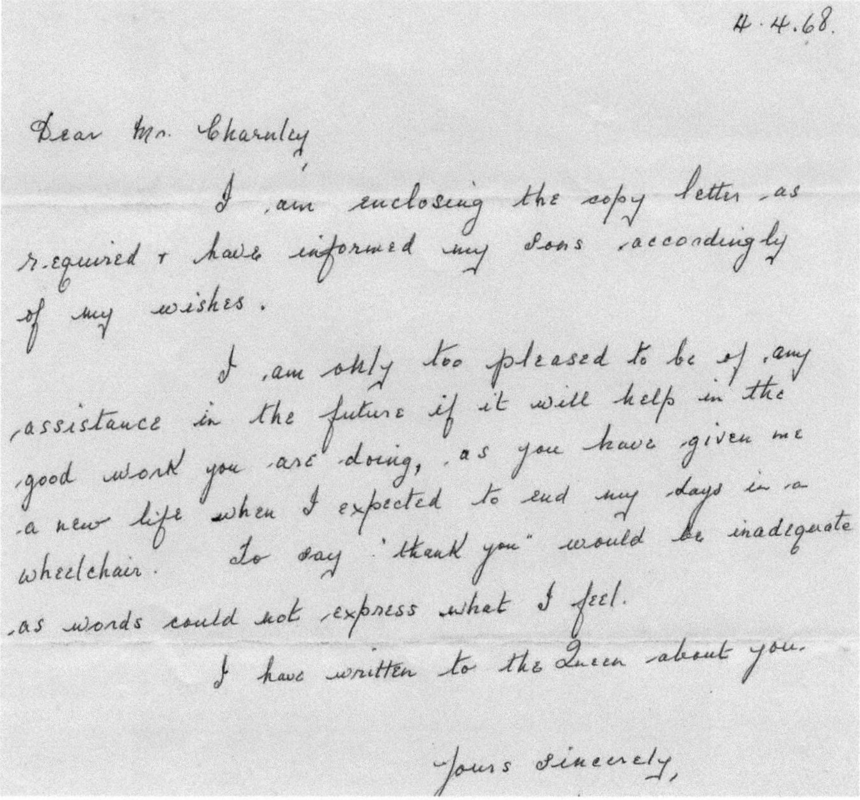

4.4.68.

Dear Mr. Charnley

I am enclosing the copy letter as required + have informed my sons accordingly of my wishes.

I am only too pleased to be of any assistance in the future if it will help in the good work you are doing, as you have given me a new life when I expected to end my days in a wheelchair. To say "thank you" would be inadequate as words could not express what I feel.

I have written to the Queen about you.

Yours sincerely,

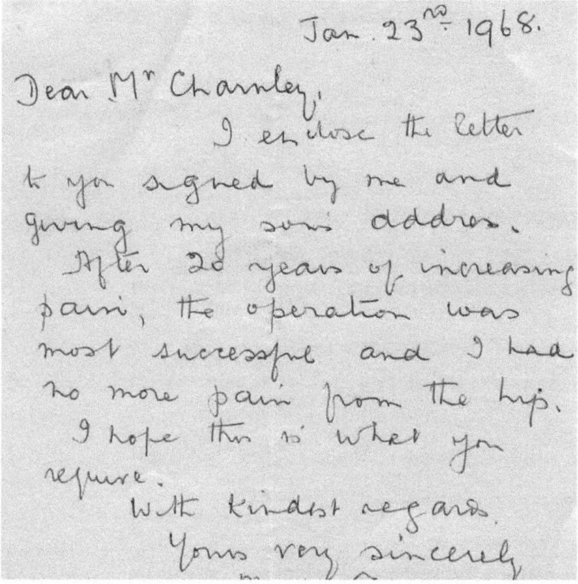

Jan. 23rd 1968.

Dear Mr Charnley,

I enclose the letter to you signed by me and giving my son's address.

After 20 years of increasing pain, the operation was most successful and I had no more pain from the hip.

I hope this is what you require.

With kindest regards.

Yours very sincerely

Figs. 3.6 and 3.7 Letters from patients to Charnley giving permission for their hip replacements to be used for medical research

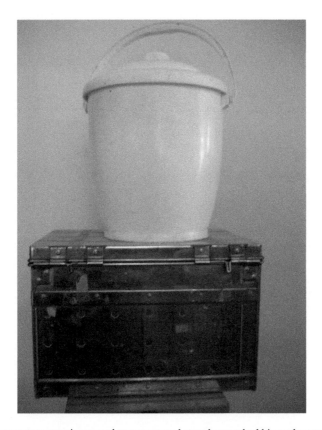

Fig. 3.8 Post mortem containers used to remove and store bequeathed hip replacements

Post-mortem Specimens

The very personal and sensitive manner in which Charnley approached the patients was very well reflected in what followed. There has never been a single complaint from the relatives. Even years after the study was completed it was not unusual to receive messages about the availability of further material from a recently deceased relative.

When the project was nearing completion 78 hips, retrieved from 57 patients, were available for the study. Majority of specimens, 44, were from female patients, while 13 were from male patients. This is a reflection of the clinical practice and the demand for the operation. Technical details of the preparation of the specimens for histological examination, as well as the interpretation of the various appearances, are outside the scope of this brief record.

The examination of the post-mortem specimens was completed by Professor Archie Malcolm under the sponsorship of the John Charnley Trust set up by Lady Charnley. The reader must refer to the original publications [2–10] on the subject.

Correlation Between the Radiographic Appearances, Histology of the Bone-Cement Interface of the Cup and the Clinical Results

There are certain aspects concerning the information derived from the study that for various reasons, have not been documented before.

These concern the correlation between the clinical results, as derived from the follow-up records, radiographic appearances of the bone-cement interface of the cup as observed on the final follow-up radiographs, and the histology of the bone-cement interface of the cup.

For the purpose of these particular studies 39 of the 78 specimens available had to be excluded. The reasons for exclusion are detailed in Table 3.4

The details of the clinical results were extracted from the records made at the last follow-up, graded for pain, function and movement according to d'Aubigne and Postel classification [11] as modified by Charnley [12].

All the radiographs were examined jointly by Professor R S M Ling OBE, FRCS, Mr M W J Older FRCS and Professor B M Wroblewski. The appearances were classified according to Hodgkinson et al. [13] and consensus was achieved in each and every case.

The Results

The 39 hips were from 30 patients; 29 from 21 females (8 bilateral) and 10 from 8 males (2 bilateral). The mean age at surgery for the whole group was 68 years 7 months (46 years 8 months – 80 years) and the mean weight 62 kg (37–87).

The underlying hip pathology was primary osteoarthritis in 25, Rheumatoid arthritis in 10, Idiopathic protrusio in 2, Paget's disease and congenital dysplasia – 1 each.

One hip had been operated upon previously by intertrochanteric osteotomy.

The mean follow-up was 5 years and 9 months (8 months to 14 years 5 months) while the time between the last follow-up and death was 1 year 11 months (2 weeks to 5 years 6 months).

Table 3.4 Exclusions from the study

22	Cemented stems with press-fit metal backed cup
6	Radiolucent cement used for both the cup and the stem
5	Revisions from Teflon to UHMWPE cups
5	Specimens previously sectioned for histology
1	McKee metal on metal arthroplasty

Clinical Results

These are shown graphically in Fig. 3.9. The most obvious feature is the severity of pain and disability of the patients accepted for the operation. Rest pain, clinically, and extensive changes radiologically, were the indications for the operation. Of the 39 hip replacements, 37 were considered to be completely pain free. Functional activity level and parameters are more difficult to assess objectively as they depend, to a large extent, on patient selection for the operation.

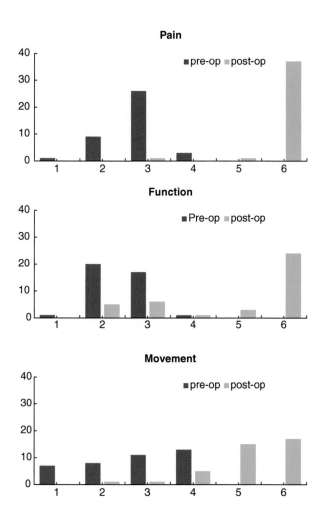

Fig. 3.9 Bar Chart showing clinical results in the post-mortem study. Before surgery and at the last follow-up before death

Radiographic Appearances and Histology of Bone-Cement Interface of the Cup

Radiographic appearances and the histology of bone cement interface was the main purpose of the study. The histological studies were carried out by Professor Archie Malcolm who suggested a classification which is shown in Table 3.5.

The correlation between the radiographic appearance according to Hodgkinson et al. [13] and histological appearances as defined by Malcolm is shown in Table 3.6.

The results of the study have shown that clinically the operation is uniformly successful. Freedom from pain is the main feature. Activity level depends on the patient selection for the operation.

Table 3.5 Histology of bone-cement interface of the cups examined. Classification suggested by Professor Malcolm and used in the study

Numerical value	Histological appearance	Fibrous membrane
0	Complete osseointegration	Nil
1	Areas of osseointegration Incomplete fibrous membrane	Incomplete
2	Complete fibrous membrane	Thin
3	- ditto -	Moderate
4	- ditto -	Thick
5	- ditto -	Gross

Table 3.6 Comparison of histological and radiographic appearances of the bone-cement interface of the cup in the 39 specimens studied

Fibrous membrane			None	Outer 3rd	Outer 3rd Mid 3rd	Complete	Socket migration
	Gross	5				x	x
	Thick	4			xx	xxxx	
	Moderate	3		xxx	xxxx	xxxx	
	Thin	2	xxx	xxxxx xxxxx	x		
	Incomplete	1	xxx xxx				
	Nil	0					
Radiographic appearance Demarcation of the socket			None	Outer 3rd	Outer 3rd Mid 3rd	Complete	Socket migration

Conclusion

From the very detailed information gathered as a result of Charnley's foresight it is clear that

– **Clinical results** do not reflect the mechanical state of the arthroplasty; there is no correlation between the radiographic appearances and the clinical results. This is not unexpected. If we assume that arthritic pain arises from the articulation then replacement of the real articulation with an artificial can be expected to offer pain relief. "Fixation" of the cup is probably less important than maintenance of the position of the cup while reducing wear to the minimum possible. (Even the metal backed press-fit cups offered freedom from pain).
– **Histology of the bone-cement** interface of the cup reflects the radiographic appearances quite accurately. Total osseointegration was not found in any of the cases, although areas of osseointegration were found in six hips where bone-cement demarcation was incomplete [10].

It could be argued that lack of total osseointegration is an indication of failure. This may be considered to be correct if the objective was to achieve osseointegration. This could only be so on the assumption that osseointegration is essential for clinical success. This assumption, however, cannot be correct. There is no correlation between the clinical results and the radiographic appearances or the histological findings; osseointegration of the cup is not essential for clinical success.

(The metal backed press-fit cups were introduced because of the demarcation of the bone-cement interface observed in some cases. Osseointegration could not have occurred – yet clinical results were successful – some over many years (Figs. 3.2, 3.3 and 3.4). The method was abandoned because of cup tilting and dislocation, not because of pain.)

The explanation must be that osseointegration is not essential for clinical success, maintenance of the position of the cup however, is essential.

It is the change in cup position resulting in a progressive loss of bone stock, that becomes an indication for revision.

It is in this context that the low frictional torque principle in Charnley hip replacement allows excellent function over so many years. It is the progressive cup penetration leading to impingement of the neck of the stem on the rim of the cup, as well as the increase in the frictional torque, that set the limit on the success of this type of surgery.

Although clinical results remain the essential part of clinical practice, radiographic appearances are a better indication of the mechanical state of the arthroplasty.

Follow-up of patients must include radiographs; verbal or written information is not adequate for the assessment of the mechanical results of hip replacement surgery.

It is essential to distinguish between the clinical success of an operation for an individual patient and the long-term success of the method of surgery.

References

1. Wroblewski BM, Fleming PA, Hall RM, Siney PD. Stem fixation in the Charnley low friction arthroplasty in young patients using an intramedullary bone block. J Bone Joint Surg (Br). 1998;80-B:273–8.
2. Follaci FM, Charnley J. A comparison of the results of femoral head prosthesis with and without cement. Clin. Orthop. 1969;62:156–61.
3. Charnley J, Follacci FM, Hammond BT. The long-term reaction of bone to self-curing acrylic cement. J Bone Joint Surg (Br). 1968;50-B:821–9.
4. Charnley J. The reaction of bone to self-curing acrylic cement. A long-term histological study in man. J Bone Joint Surg (Br). 1970;52-B:340–53.
5. Charnley J. Acrylic cement in orthopaedic surgery. London: Edinburgh; 1970.
6. Charnley J. Low-friction arthroplasty of the hip. Theory and practice. Berlin: Springer; 1979. p. 25–40.
7. Malcolm AJ. Pathology of cemented low-friction arthroplasties in autopsy specimens. In: Older J, editor. Implant bone interface. London: Springer; 1990. p. 77–81.
8. Malcolm AJ. Bone-implant interface in long-standing prosthetic implants. In: Langlais F, Tomens B, editors. Major reconstructions in oncologic and non-tumoral conditions. Berlin: Springer; 1991. p. 319–28.
9. Willert HG, Buchhorn GH. Histological analysis of interface. In: Learmonth ID, editor. Interfaces in total hip arthroplasty. London: Springer; 2000.
10. Draenert K, Draenert Y. Properties of bone cement: the three interfaces. In: Breush–Malchau, editors. The well cemented total hip arthroplasty. Theory and practice. Springer; 2005. p. 93–107.
11. d'Aubigne MR, Postel M. Functional results of hip arthroplasty with acrylic prosthesis. J Bone Joint Surg (Am). 1954;36-A:451–75.
12. Charnley J. The long-term results of low-friction arthroplasty of the hip as primary intervention. J Bone Joint Surg. 1972;54-B:61–76.
13. Hodgkinson JP, Shelley P, Wroblewski BM. The correlation between the roentgenographic appearance and operative findings at the bone-cement junction of the socket in Charnley low-friction arthroplasties. Clin Orthop. 1988;228:105–9.

Chapter 4
Clinical Results

The clinical results of this operation are so good that one often feels they are too good to be true.

The driving force behind the development of total hip arthroplasty was Charnley's desire to help patients disabled by painful arthritic hips. The surgical procedures available: intertrochanteric osteotomy, arthrodesis, or excision – pseudarthrosis – did not offer predictably significant clinical benefit; and if they did it was only limited and in a carefully selected minority.

It is interesting that pain, hip pain, the main indication for surgery, has received so little detailed attention. True enough, every assessment scoring system includes pain – even at times using visual analogue scale – but none define hip pain.

At some stage on the "patient pathway" and almost certainly very early on – and maybe even before the patient is seen – an assumption is made that the problem is "a painful hip". Very often the radiograph is seen before the patient becomes the focus of attention.

Deep seated structures, when affected by a disease process, do not offer localising symptoms – certainly not initially. It is generally assumed that pain from an arthritic joint arises in the worn arthritic joint surfaces. After all, an intra-articular injection of local anaesthetic offers immediate relief of pain. What about the capsule? At some stage it was considered the source of pain and the cause of fixed deformities. Excision of the capsule has never been the part of the Charnley hip replacement, although some limited exposures did advocate the excision of the capsule.

The immediate relief of pain remains the driving force behind the surgery of total hip arthroplasty. The relief of pain is considered to be the success of the treatment offered. And yet, pain can only be experienced by the sufferer. Painful episodes cannot be quantified in terms that can be understood, compared with that of other sufferers or recorded in the memory for any future reference – a fortunate state for the human race.

© Springer International Publishing Switzerland 2016

B.M. Wroblewski et al., *Charnley Low-Frictional Torque Arthroplasty of the Hip: Practice and Results*, DOI 10.1007/978-3-319-21320-0_4

Any attempt to assess, record, recall or compare the results of a treatment must understand and accept the limitations. In short – pain is personal and so is the relief from it.

In clinical practice where brevity, simplicity and comparability is essential; the d'Aubigne and Postel method of assessment [1] as modified by Charnley [2] continues to be most practical. Pain relief after successful THA has practical implications for follow-up. A natural symptomatic joint, replaced with a neuropathic spacer cannot become symptomatic unless the failure involves the living structures – a late and often very late state of affairs.

Activity level achieved as a result of a successful THA is not a characteristic of a particular design, material or even a method of component fixation – certainly not in the short term – it is a reflection of patient selection for the operation. Activity level advertises success, attracts would be candidates some of whom may have unreasonable expectations.

Single case success is attractive both clinically and commercially – a most unfortunate combination.

It is interesting how the range of hip movement has received little attention. Freedom from pain need not be accompanied by full range of hip movements except in very exceptional cases and situations.

In preoperative assessment, patient selection and identification of the source and severity of the problem is most essential. At follow-up comparison of serial radiographs is mandatory.

Clinical Assessment

Successful clinical results uncovered the demand and extended the indications for the operation. Pressure of numbers and the increasing costs focused the attention on the financial implications. Initially the operation was used as a "unit of currency" against which the cost of other procedures was assessed. More recently the cost-benefit ratio, for individual patients, expressed as "quality of life", is becoming the standard. This is not unexpected. Pain – hip pain – is not immediately obvious to an observer. Furthermore, severity of pain does not usually leave a permanent imprint on our memory – fortunately.

Restriction of movement or activity may be more obvious but only to those close by. Activity level, achieved as the result of freedom from pain, becomes clear for all to see without the need for explanation or comment.

Thus hip pain, the indication for the operation is quickly forgotten, while activity level advertises individual clinical success and becomes the target for would be patients to aim for.

The indications for the operation and the patients expectations have moved away from pain relief to expected activity level.

In clinical practice viewing of radiographs often comes before clinical assessment. In this context the term: "end-stage arthritis" is becoming common; a most unfortunate development. It is not only unscientific but full of emotional overtones. History and examination must come first. A radiograph shows me what the hip looks like but the patient tells me what it feels like!

History

Patients presenting for consideration of hip replacement surgery are often "self-selected" and maybe even "self referred." They may already have a record of previous consultations. More often than not they may have preconceived ideas as to what benefits are to be had from a successful hip replacement. It has been observed over the past 40 years or so that the type of patient has gradually changed. In the 1970s patients often presented late in the disease process. Pain was often severe, disability great, deformities marked, dependence on sticks or crutches common. Then followed a period when patients presented with fears of "being confined to a wheelchair". More recently high expectations are the order of the day. Why this changing pattern? Confidence and familiarity and unreasonable claims of success – often based on the very early "single case success stories" may be some of the reasons.

Detailed history is essential and must follow a clearly set pattern no matter that the problem and the decision as to treatment are immediately obvious. By the time the patient enters the consulting room every opportunity must be taken to establish a relationship which may be for a lifetime – either of each other or of the arthroplasty.

Time of onset and duration of symptoms, pain patterns, its effect on daily activities, patient's understanding of the problem, but above all knowledge of the disease process, the likely progress and finally the ins and outs of surgery. After physical examination, then and only then, should the radiograph be viewed. It is not the purpose of this work to spell basic details of history taking and examination.

Young patient, long history, would suggest congenital problems. Female patient with restriction of all movements apart for flexion – probably protrusio. Muscular male with a history of sporting activity – could be slipped upper femoral epiphysis. Grumbling pain with full movements of the hip, be on the lookout for avascular necrosis. Sudden "collapse" rare – beware of something unusual or even sinister here, special investigations may be indicated.

Be on the lookout for leg length discrepancy. Disease process – other than protrusio or early AVN – should result in limb shortening. Apparent limb lengthening, of which the patient is invariably unaware, indicates early arthritis with a well preserved proximal lever, femoral head contained within the acetabulum.

Beware of fixed pelvic obliquity due to long standing spinal problems. All problems may not be solved by THA and leg lengthening after surgery will be bitterly complained of. First consultation need not lead to surgery.

A word of warning about a congenital dislocation of the hip with secondary degenerative changes, **adduction deformity** and symptoms severe enough to warrant surgery. The contralateral hip dysplasia may not be obvious because of the pelvic obliquity. Successful hip replacement "uncovers" the dysplastic hip, arthritic changes – now symptomatic – may follow rather quickly. What must not be forgotten with limb length discrepancy is that the knee on the longer side functions in flexion, degenerative changes of the knee may follow. The knee on the side of the adducted hip functions in valgus. Levelling of the pelvis after THA exaggerates the valgus of the knee which makes walking difficult.

Pain severe enough may make or break an individual, yet how quickly it is forgotten. The hip joint so deeply seated has not often been studied as a source of pain. The patterns presented are so varied that an attempt was made to establish a more detailed description. The areas of the anatomy are shown in Fig. 4.1. It is this variable pattern, without sensory or neuromuscular involvement that is typical.

Grading Method for Pain, Function and Movement in the Hip

Charnley adopted the grading method of d'Aubigne and Postel (1954) [1] with modifications [2] to record pain, function and movement in the hip, both pre-operatively and at follow-up (Fig. 4.2, Table 4.1). The method is simple, clear, not time consuming but demands some clarification.

Pain

Assessment for pain is probably best carried out by comparison of the extremes:

Grades 1–6, 2–5 with the 3–4 "grey area" where significant nocturnal pain is prominent in grade 3.

Grade 1 Severe spontaneous as in a fracture of the femoral neck, septic arthritis or some other more sinister pathology. Exceedingly rare in an arthritic hip. If genuinely so severe caution must be the byword – be aware and seek other problems to be addressed.

Grade 6 Completely pain free as in a normal hip or with an excellent result of hip replacement. It must not be forgotten that a very stiff or fused hip very often is painless.

Grade 2 Pain at rest or permitting limited activity with the use of support – a walking frame, sticks or crutches, with frequent resort to analgesics. Patients experience pain virtually all the time but the severity may vary becoming severe when precipitated by sudden movement when under load: as in getting up from a sitting position, turning, climbing stairs or stumbling. Not often seen in more recent years: patients usually present much earlier.

Grade 5 No more than an occasional discomfort, settles quickly with rest, analgesics not usually taken except very occasionally. Can be regarded, and often is, as

Fig. 4.1 Distribution of pain referral areas of the anatomy

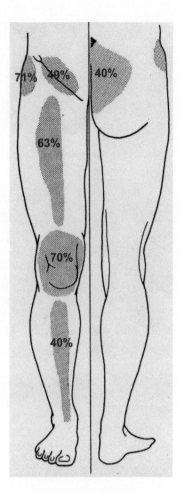

a satisfactory result of total hip arthroplasty. If presenting as symptoms of early arthritis, in the hope to achieve some unreasonable level of activity after hip replacement, caution is the watchword – possible complications must be balanced against "moving up a grade".

The 3/4 grades present the dividing line.

Grade 3 Probably the most common grade presenting for hip replacement. Being significant pain at rest – especially nocturnal. May be gleaned from the patients demeanour when giving the history: pain alters the face especially around the eyes and wipes out the sense of humour. It is the combination of pain, fear of sudden severe episodes of pain and depravation of sleep that becomes an absolute indication for hip replacement.

Grade 4 This may be considered as a borderline situation though clearly other factors must be taken into consideration. No night and only minimal rest pain. It is

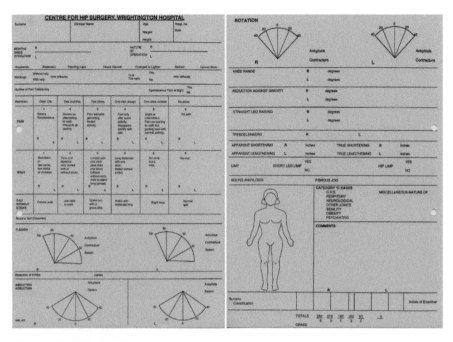

Fig. 4.2 Green Card – Charnley clinical assessment chart

Table 4.1 Charnley clinical assessment chart

Grade	Pain	Function (activity)	Movement (Total range)
1	Severe Spontaneous	Few yards or bedridden Two sticks or crutches	0–30°
2	Severe on attempting walking. Prevents all activity	Time and distance very limited with or without support	60°
3	Tolerable permitting limited Activity. Pain at rest	Limited with support, difficult without support. Able to stand for relatively long periods	100°
4	On activity settles with rest	Long distance with one stick Limited without it	160°
5	Slight, intermittent, improves with activity	No stick but limp	210°
6	Pain free	Normal	260°

this group of patients that need more time in a consultation and a single consultation may not be sufficient to make the decision. Fear of loss of independence of being confined to a wheelchair (somehow the notion of cripples and wheelchairs remains ingrained) and somehow missing an opportunity of a successful treatment is often at the back of a patients mind.

Having obtained the history and confirmed the findings on examination, and having explained the radiographic appearances, the need is to explain the pattern into which the whole picture fits. Patients have no maps or charts against which to place themselves or their hip problems. We all tend to selectively pick out what we want to hear, or accept only the result that would be in our interest, there must be something of an optimistic gambler in us all.

Time spent on a consultation, especially the first one, is never and should never be wasted. A good rapport becomes even more important years later.

Function/Activity

Assessment of function before, and even more so after hip replacement is a very complex task and no method can be satisfactory to all. Attempts have been made to bring in various activities as an aid in assessing this parameter. The best example of complexity of the subject can be seen when contemplating the Olympic Games: numerous disciplines, numerous competitors, fractions of units separating competitors, only one winner – yet each one attempting to assess "activity". How can a clinician attempt to define or describe and put on record details for an individual patient? It cannot be some rigid system, divorced from the individual, or based on some arbitrary scale. Function is personal to the individual. It cannot and must not be a desire for some unfulfilled expectations from the past or hopes for the future. It is here that the guiding role of the surgeon is so important. A balance must be struck between what is possible, desirable and what can be achieved – barring complications. Temptation of extrapolating from the last successful case must be tempered with caution.

Grades 1–6

Grade 1 Confined to bed, wheelchair, certainly confined and housebound. Very dependent on others for activities even in and around the house. Unusual with just a single arthritic hip, most likely with multiple joints being involved e.g. rheumatoid arthritis.

Grade 6 Normal for age and gender which clearly is a vast range, not only of abilities, but also of needs and expectations

Grade 2 Permitting limited, independent activity, slow with difficulty and with support.

Grade 5 Just short of normal, yet very good. This grade and limit gradually creeps up on all of us. It is here that a sudden burst of activity may lead to undesirable consequences. Acceptable result of THA though at times may not be quite what the patient expected or the surgeon was hoping for. This group of patients like grade 4 may be possible to identify before surgery.

Grade 4 Mobile, even a relatively good walking distance, but a limp and use of support – a stick or a single crutch is required when outdoors. Reasonable result of THA if pain is completely relieved otherwise not a happy state of affairs.

Grade 3 Severely limited but capable of some independent outdoor activities although always in need of support. May be a good guide for the acceptance for THA but not a good result of the failed operation. If pain is relieved, as at times following removal of the artificial joint, that limitation of activities may just be accepted even if not exactly acceptable.

Grading of activity both before and after surgery may at times include daily activities common to all, or specific to the individual patient. The list can be expanded or limited but should include activities common to all of us i.e. dressing, undressing, walking, climbing stairs, hygiene or even recreational activities such as distance walking, dancing or some sporting activities. (This last group brings us closer to the Olympic Games issues).

Range of Hip Movements

This was recorded by charting the position of the lower limb – with respect to the diagram – showing the range. Sum of all movements is then represented by a single number. Ankle separation, a very valuable parameter, was tape-measured. Although this parameter can be measured and recorded very objectively, the restrictions that loss of movement imposes on an individual may not be appreciated unless specific questions are posed. Again it centres around daily activities – here the ability to dress without hindrance – socks, shoes and toenails feature prominently. (Night time activities are not often mentioned in the context of hip movements).

Refinement of Assessment

Assessment of a patient's activity level after THA may not possible if there are factors other than the hip that contribute to the disability. It is primarily for that reason that Charnley suggested the modification with the addition of the prefixes **A**, **B** **or C**.

Prefix A: Would indicate the patient with a unilateral hip problem with no other factors, mechanical or medical, that would affect mobility. This is the group that can be used for the purpose of assessing activity level after hip replacement.

Prefix B: Bilateral hip involvement in the disease process but no other factors affecting mobility.

Prefix C: Unilateral or bilateral hip involvement with other pathologies, mechanical or medical, affecting mobility. In this group would be patients with rheumatoid arthritis, cardiac or pulmonary problems, general debility or gross obesity. Under such circumstances pain relief and improvements in the range of movements would be possible to assess after surgery, but the operation, even if successful could not be used to assess improvement of function/activity.

In clinical practice a number of issues became apparent. Only patients in group **A** could provide a measure of success of the operation in terms of activity. In group **C** the only parameters that could be assessed was pain relief and range of movements of the hip joint. Although individual patients were in a position to express their opinion in terms of improvement of function, their results could never match the patients in category **A**. Patients in category **B**, and with bilateral hip arthroplasties, hopefully successful, could gauge the level of improvement in function but only against their previous level.

No patient could be upgraded to the level above their original grade, no matter how successful the hip replacement had been. With time there would be an expected reduction in the numbers in category **A** and an increase in the categories **B** and **C**.

Increasing follow-up would also expose the arthroplasty, in the **A** category patients, to the highest activity level. Thus, any attempt to assess the results would have to take these aspects into consideration.

When assessing the long-term results it is very interesting to observe changing patterns. Reduction in the percentage in the group **A** and increase in the group **B** clearly indicates the increasing numbers of patients having bilateral THA. Change from **A** and **B** to **C** group would indicate an increasing proportion of patients with multiple disabilities - making general statements concerning assessment of function less valuable.

This relatively simple and easy to follow system has advantages which may not be immediately obvious. The visual scale, the movement, hopefully from low to high figures is an easy to understand scale and an excellent mode to break down the problem into three understandable parameters – accepting that assessing function will always be subjective and more likely for anecdotal presentation being taken advantage of.

The drawbacks of the classification. No indication is given of fixed deformities or whether the problem is bilateral hip disease, or arthroplasties, or indeed, a mixture of both.

Because of the large numbers of patients undergoing hip replacement it was considered, correctly, that compliance with any method of assessment and documentation would be inversely proportional to its complexity. The d'Aubigne and Postel system [1] as modified by Lazansky and Charnley [2] became the standard. In time, with increasing follow-up and experience, there arose a need to expand the methods of assessment of functional results. The advent of sophisticated methods of measuring wear – as in joint simulators – stimulated research in an attempt to bring the clinical and experimental methods closer for the purpose of comparison. If patients' activity levels could be expressed in purely mechanical parameters, as used experimentally, then testing of new materials could be carried out, at least initially, without the need for patient involvement.

Other methods of assessment are frequently being used. Complexity may imply quality but percentage figures do not convey the percentage of which parameter. In the same context "quality of life" comes into prominence. This parameter, although often quoted in an affluent society, has no great value in the context of clinical result. In fact, it can be argued, that with some communities starving while others watch commercials advertising low-calorie diets, 'quality of life' measures are best avoided.

Although pre and post-operative detailed assessment and recording are essential and form a part of good clinical practice, it must be pointed out that any method may become a measure of patient selection and not a measure of the result of the operation. THA is such a consistently excellent procedure that what is being assessed is whether the indications for selecting the patient were adequate.

With increasing follow-up clinical assessment loses its importance – except for the patients with the longest and ever increasing follow-up. The patterns of failure pave the way for evidence based improvements. We must distinguish between clinical success of the operation for an individual patient and the long-term success of the method.

References

1. d'Aubigne MR, Postel M. Functional results of hip arthroplasty with acrylic prosthesis. J Bone Joint Surg (Am). 1954;36-A:451–75.
2. Charnley J. The long-term results of low-friction arthroplasty of the hip as primary intervention. J Bone Joint Surg. 1972;54-B:61–76.

Chapter 5
Leg Over-Lengthening After Total Hip Arthroplasty Identification of Patients at Risk

Leg length discrepancy, in general, and leg over-lengthening in particular, after total hip arthroplasty, has emerged as a topic of interest and dissatisfaction. In some quarters leg over-lengthening has been quoted as a common cause for litigation [1, 2]. "Limb lengthening is not uncommon after total hip replacement and may cause subjective problems for patients … 27 % of patients required heel lifts on the un-operated side" [3]. Leg length inequality "… as a cause of aseptic loosening, and unexplained pain, warrants investigation in THA patients" [4]. The high rate of dissatisfaction among patients with leg length inequality and the untoward results associated with this inequality, indicate that surgeons performing THA should familiarise themselves with a reliable method of equalising leg lengths intra-operatively" [5].

Ranawat and Rodriguez [6] attempted to assess functional leg length inequality (FLLI) by reviewing their records and gaining a response from the Hip Society members hoping to establish prevalence, aetiology and management. Fourteen percent of patients were noted to have pelvic obliquity and FLLI one month after surgery – all resolving by 6 months. Among the causes suggested by the respondents were: tightness of the periarticular tissues with resultant pelvic obliquity and degenerative conditions of the spine [6]. The direction of the pelvic obliquity, whether towards or away from the affected hip, was not stated. Reference to "tightness of the periarticular tissues" [6] and the fact that a proportion of patients needed a heel lift on the un-operated side [3] suggests that the tilt referred to was towards the symptomatic side thus highlighting abduction deformity of the osteoarthritic hip and functional limb lengthening on the symptomatic, arthritic side.

Despite the demand for THA the deformities associated with the arthritic hip have not received much attention. Lloyd-Roberts [7] in his Robert Jones Lecture suggested that fixed deformities in osteoarthritis of the hip are "due to capsular shortening reinforced by reflex guarding in the muscles supplied by the motor branches of the sensory nerves to the lower part of the cavity – such as pectineus, quadratus femoris and the adductor group". This dynamic deformity was later followed by a structural deformity from the fibrosis of the musculo-tendinous function. Lloyd-Roberts felt that osteophytes, once developed, were unlikely to prevent movement by interlocking growth [7].

© Springer International Publishing Switzerland 2016
B.M. Wroblewski et al., *Charnley Low-Frictional Torque Arthroplasty of the Hip: Practice and Results*, DOI 10.1007/978-3-319-21320-0_5

Pearson and Ridell [8] divided idiopathic osteoarthritic hips into two groups: the adducted and the non-adducted variety suggesting that muscle spasm was the primary cause, the final position depending on capsular contracture. (Mechanically these changes cannot develop in an ambulant patient, against gravity and deficient proximal lever – head and neck). Abduction deformity of a normal hip has been described with fibrous bands of genetic origin [9–11] or following intra-muscular injections [12]. The abducted position of the hip, usually with flexion and external rotation, is well recognised in acute poliomyelitis.

Why has the problem emerged after over 40 years of hip replacement surgery? Can the pitfalls be anticipated and, if not avoided, at least better understood and explained before surgery?

Patient Selection

Strict criteria of patient selection was the essential aspect in the evolution of the Charnley hip replacement. Significant pain at rest, failure of all conservative measures and an often radiologically destroyed hip, were the indications for hip arthroplasty. True limb shortening was, almost always, a part of the clinical picture. Radiologically upper pole grade III changes was the common finding [13]. The benefit of immediate pain relief far outweighed any possible disadvantage of failure to restore leg length. When this was achieved it was considered a bonus. So what has changed? Increasing experience with this type of surgery has led to an extension of the indications, increased the demand and higher patient expectations.

The term "end stage arthritis" has gained popularity but failed to define the clinical problem or the radiographic morphology of the osteoarthritic hip [13].

Surgical Technique

Limited exposures, excision of the capsule, laxity of the joint at trial reduction and the fear of post-operative dislocation all contribute to tight reduction – under anaesthetic. This is equated with stability – unfortunately at the expense of limb lengthening. Could this be avoided? Probably.

Excision of the Capsule

Excision of the capsule has never been a part of the Charnley technique. In fact preservation of the capsule was the teaching, and for very good reason. The hip capsule is not the site of the pain. Exposure, by trochanteric osteotomy, gives full access: a circumferential view of the acetabulum and access to the medullary canal. Checking stability at trial reduction, by joint distraction, offers a very definite endpoint. Excision of the capsule exposes the muscles which, under anaesthetic, allow a fair degree of stretch. This elastic "give" has no definite end-point, hence the need for lengthening, by component selection, and limb over-lengthening. Overstretching the muscles will lead to loss of proprioception, and even loss of power. Combined with the neuropathic nature of arthroplasty over-lengthening, laxity and muscle weakness would be opposite to the initial goal.

Component Selection

Pre-operative planning should include component selection as well as the detail of their positioning in relation to radiographic landmarks. With standard monoblock Charnley stem and the selection of mainly two cup sizes, the planning was focused on the details of the surgical technique. Modularity, although offering a wide choice, may result in the postponement of the decision until the final stage of the operation when both the cup and the stem are already securely fixed. The only remaining option will be the seating of the modular head on the neck taper. It is at this stage that leg length inequality, over-lengthening, may be the inevitable result.

Arthroplasty Technique

The advent of "minimally invasive" techniques and "resurfacing" must be considered. The techniques demand, ideally, anatomically intact, near normal geometry of the hip joint where limb shortening is not a problem, in fact in the early stages of arthritis, apparent, functional limb lengthening may be present. Maintaining limb length equality may be a problem and lengthening may result.

Patients at Risk for Limb Over-Lengthening

What has not received detailed attention is our ability to identify patients at risk for limb over-lengthening. Although anticipating the problem may not always be the solution, understanding the problem is the essential part of pre-operative planning and the informed consent.

Theoretical Considerations

With any painful condition it is natural to seek a position of comfort. In order to reduce the load on a painful hip, while standing, the pelvis is tilted to the symptomatic side, the hip is abducted, externally rotated, and the knee flexed. The contralateral hip, must of necessity, be adducted (observe Michelangelo's David). While walking the body weight is moved over the symptomatic hip – reducing the load and the pain. These postural characteristics can only be adopted if certain mechanical features are present.

1. Intact proximal lever. The arthritic hip must have the proximal lever, head and neck, relatively intact and contained with a normal or near normal acetabulum, allowing unhindered abduction movement. The radiographic appearances can be anticipated: incipient type arthritis, upper pole grade I and II, concentric, protrusio or medial pole type. Upper pole grade III type would be rare [13]. Inferior, medial osteophyte, "the head drop" is typical.
2. The contralateral hip must allow adduction movement and thus be normal, near normal or be fixed in an adducted position.
3. The spine must be mobile to compensate for the pelvic tilt. Alternatively, a fixed lateral spinal deformity, resulting in pelvic obliquity will be the primary cause of limb length inequality. The history of spinal problems should alert the surgeon to the possibility of functional limb length inequality, while the limb inequality and pelvic tilt should alert the surgeon to the likelihood of spinal problems.
4. Soft tissue, capsular, contractures and osteophyte formation, must be secondary.

Clinical Relevance of Theoretical Considerations

With the information in mind it is possible to identify patients who are at risk for leg over-lengthening as a result of THA

Measurement of Limb Length Discrepancy

True and apparent leg length discrepancy (LLD) was measured by the standard, clinical methods. It was felt, however, that a functional leg length discrepancy (FLLD) would be of practical interest, because this is the discrepancy that affects patient's gait and indicates the need and the extent of the footwear build-up (Figs. 5.1 and 5.2).

This measurement is taken with the patient erect. Theoretical considerations suggest that patients at risk for post-operative leg over-lengthening are those with pre-operative abduction deformity of the hip.

We defined the abduction deformity as being present when the symptomatic hip functioned or had become fixed in a position lateral to the anatomical.

Radiographic morphology of both hips was recorded and radiographs of the spine were taken if indicated. Our findings are the result of examination of 5,000 patients presenting for Charnley LFA.

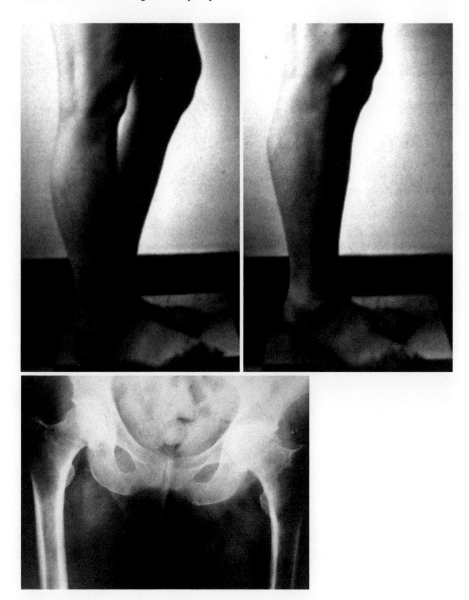

Figs. 5.1 and 5.2 Functional leg lengthening: abducted left hip, knee in flexion. With the knee extended right heel is off the ground. Radiograph shows pelvic tilt to the left side, well preserved proximal lever (head and neck) large infero-medial, "head drop" osteophyte – opposite hip normal

The Incidence

We identified 182 patients with abduction deformity – an incidence of 3.64 %. There were 80 males and 102 females, their mean age was 63 years (20–80 years).

Pelvic Tilt

Pelvic tilt towards the symptomatic side was the typical finding as was expected from theoretical considerations. However, a small group of patients with <u>bilateral</u> abduction deformity was identified (Fig. 5.6). In this group the pelvis was level.

Aetiology

Two aetiological groups: primary and secondary, abduction deformity, were identi-fied. The characteristic features are outlined in Tables 5.1 and 5.2 and Figs. 5.3, 5.4, 5.5, 5.6, 5.7, 5.8 and 5.9.

Of the 192 hips, 23 (12.6 %) had been operated upon before. Of the remaining 169, 152 (90 %) showed an intact proximal lever making an abducted position pos-sible. Only 17: 10 % showed upper pole Grade III changes (Table 5.3).

Table 5.1 Abduction deformity of osteoarthritic hips: aetiological groups. Other than primary bilateral all had a pelvic obliquity towards the symptomatic side

Primary	Unilateral	Affecting single hip
		Opposite hip normal, near normal or fixed in an adducted position
		Pelvic tilt towards the affected arthritic hip
	Bilateral	Both hips in abducted position
		Fixed external rotation of both hips
		Pelvis level
Secondary	Post surgery	Resulting directly from an operative treatment of an osteoarthritic hip
	Post traumatic	Resulting from non-operative treatment of the hip joint
	Spinal	Abduction deformity with a pelvic tilt secondary to a fixed spinal deformity
	Mixed	Having features of two or more of the secondary groups

Table 5.2 The incidence of abduction deformity in 5,000 patients presenting for LFA

| | | Number of patients | Incidence % | Gender | | Age | |
				Male	Female	Years	Range
Primary	Unilateral	130	2.6	54	76	67	28–80
	Bilateral	10	0.2	5	5	55	44–67
Secondary	Post surgery	23	0.46	11	12	58	20–79
	Post traumatic	10	0.2	7	3	50	25–72
	Spinal	6	0. 12	2	4	58	40–70
	Mixed	3	0.06	1	2	57	48–69
Total		182	3.64	80	102	63	20.80

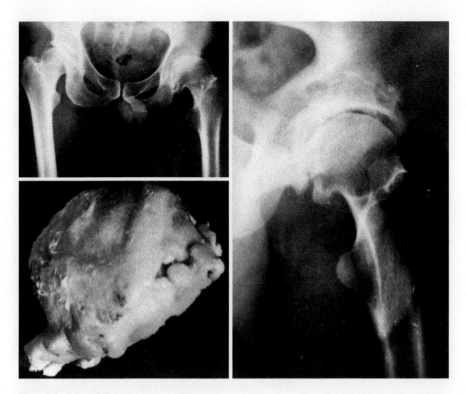

Figs. 5.3, 5.4 and 5.5 Primary, unilateral. Note pelvic tilt to the affected side and the inferior osteophyte

Comparison of Limb Lengths

Comparison of limb lengths – functional, real or apparent is only possible if the contralateral hip is radiologically normal. Of this large group of 5000 patients, only 70: 1.4 % were truly at risk for post-operative limb lengthening. The discrepancy measured 3.2 cm mean (range 0.7–5 cm) (Table 5.4).

Understanding the importance of leg length discrepancy in general, and leg lengthening after THA in particular, is important for a number of specific reasons.

Clinical Awareness

Clinical experience suggests that patients are rarely aware of apparent or real leg lengthening before surgery. The explanation is probably relatively simple. Abducted position is a position of rest, reduced load and comfort, therefore, less likely to be the subject of a complaint. Pain free, mobile hip with leg lengthening results in a

Fig. 5.6 Bilaterally
abducted hip, pelvis level.
Note patient's posture.
Passage through a door
only by a sideway shuffle

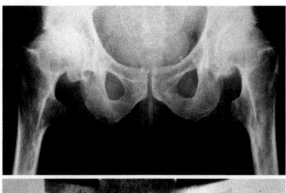
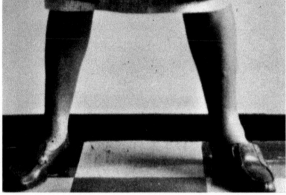

pelvic tilt which may cause backache, but also creates a sense of instability when standing on the longer leg.

Patients are more likely to accept a built up shoe because full leg length could not be restored by THA; they are certainly less likely to accept a built up shoe on the unoperated, normal side.

Clinical examination will alert the surgeon to the possibility of the post-operative limb lengthening in this group of patients. The incidence will almost certainly increase as patients with early changes and higher expectations are accepted for surgery. The problems will be further exacerbated by limited exposures, soft tissue, capsular excision and insistence of tight reduction of the hip joint.

Figs. 5.7 and 5.8 Post traumatic: arthritis. Original injury treated by single leg traction

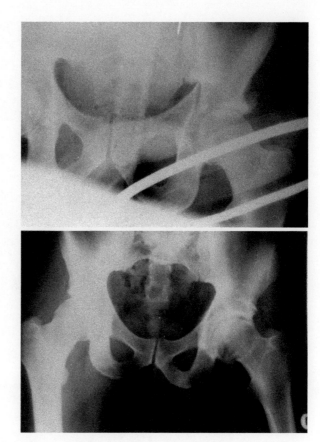

It may be of interest to point out that during the 48 year experience with the Charnley LFA (1962–2011) there has never been a revision carried out for limb over-lengthening, neither has there been a case of litigation.

In summary: The surgery of hip replacement can be considered as a three stage clinical practice:

1st Selection of **patients** for surgery.
2nd Surgery on **the hip**.
3rd The follow-up: 'after sales' surveillance of the **implant**.

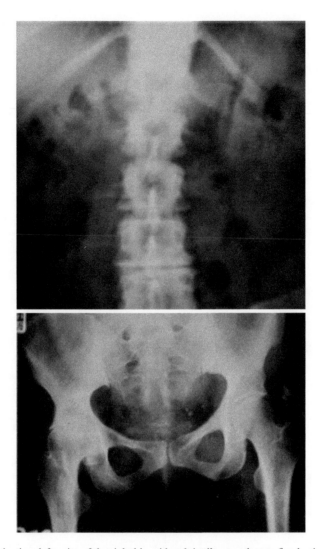

Fig. 5.9 Abduction deformity of the right hip with pelvic tilt secondary to fixed spinal deformity

Table 5.3 Radiographic morphology of the abducted arthritic hip – excluding post-surgery cases (Bilateral cases – 10 patients: 20 hips)

		Number	Incipient	Upper pole I, II and III	Concentric	Protrusio	Medial pole
Primary	Unilateral	130	8	57	13	28	15	9
	Bilateral	20	0	14	0	2	2	2
Secondary	Post traumatic	10	0	4	2	4	0	0
	Spinal	6	0	1	2	3	0	0
	Mixed	3	2	0	0	0	0	1
Total		169	10	76	17	37	17	12

Table 5.4 Limb length discrepancy when contralateral hip was radiologically normal

		Number of patients	No leg length discrepancy	Functional shortening	Functional lengthening
Primary	Unilateral	51	12	0	39
Secondary	Post surgery	7	3	0	4
	Post traumatic	6	0	0	6
	Spinal	3	0	0	3
	Mixed	3	0	0	3
Total		70	15	0	55

References

1. White AB. Study probes closed claim causes. AAOS: Bulletin. 1994;26–7.
2. Hoffman AA, Skrzynski MC. Leg length inequality and nerve palsy in total hip replacement: a lawyer awaits! Orthopaedics. 2000;23:943–4.
3. Williamson JA, Redding FW. Limb length discrepancy and related problems following total hip joint replacement. Clin Orthop. 1978;134:135–8.
4. Turula KB, Friesberg O, Lindholm TS, Tallroth K, Vankka E. Leg length inequality after total hip arthroplasty. Clin Orthop. 1986;202:163–8.
5. Edeen J, Sharkey PF, Alexander AH. Clinical significance of leg length inequality after total hip arthroplasty. Am J Orthop. 1995;24(4):347–51.
6. Ranawat CS, Rodriguez JA. Functional leg length inequality following total hip arthroplasty. J Arthroplasty. 1997;12(4):359–64.
7. Lloyd-Roberts GC. The role of capsular changes in osteoarthritis of the hip. J Bone Joint Surg Br. 1955;37:8–47.
8. Pearson JR, Riddell DW. Idiopathic osteoarthritis of the hip. Ann Rheum Dis. 1962;21:31–9.
9. Mehta MH. Bilateral congenital contracture of the ilio-tibial tract. J Bone Joint Surg Br. 1972;54:532–4.
10. Wolbrink AJ, Hsu Z, Bianco AJ. Abduction contracture of shoulders and hips secondary to fibrous bands. J Bone Joint Surg Am. 1973;55:844–6.
11. Shen Young-Shung. Abduction contracture of the hip in children. J Bone Joint Surg Br. 1975;57:483.
12. De Valderrama JAF. The cause of limited flexion adduction of the hip in children. J Bone Joint Surg Br. 1970;52:179.
13. Wroblewski BM, Charnley J. Radiographic morphology of the osteoarthritic hip. J Bone Joint Surg Br. 1982;64:568–9.

Chapter 6
Radiographic Assessment of the Osteoarthritic Hip

Detailed documentation forms an integral part of pre-operative assessment. Unfortunately this aspect is not often brought up as part of the more general teaching or practical management of a patient's problem, unless it presents an unusual appearance or a diagnostic riddle. Any method of assessment or documentation must not be so detailed as to be time consuming, or so vague as to be of little value.

Radiographic assessment needs to be made in two parts: The underlying hip pathology and the radiographic appearance of the arthritic hip. The first will give some indication of the underlying general problems, the second the radiographic appearances as this may have a bearing on the technique of hip replacement. The classification originally proposed by Charnley serves well and requires minimum of time yet offers essential basic information (Fig. 6.1).

Osteoarthritis:	
Primary	Mono and bi-articular
	Poly-articular (GOA) [generalised osteoarthritis]
Secondary	Congenital dysplasia/subluxation/dislocation
	Perthe's disease
	Slipped upper femoral epiphysis
	Trauma
	Fractured femoral neck
	Sepsis – acute
	Sepsis – chronic
	Quadrantic head necrosis (cause if known or suspected)
Rheumatoid arthritis	
Ankylosing spondylitis	
Paget's disease	
Protrusio acetabuli	
Unclassified	

© Springer International Publishing Switzerland 2016
B.M. Wroblewski et al., *Charnley Low-Frictional Torque Arthroplasty of the Hip: Practice and Results*, DOI 10.1007/978-3-319-21320-0_6

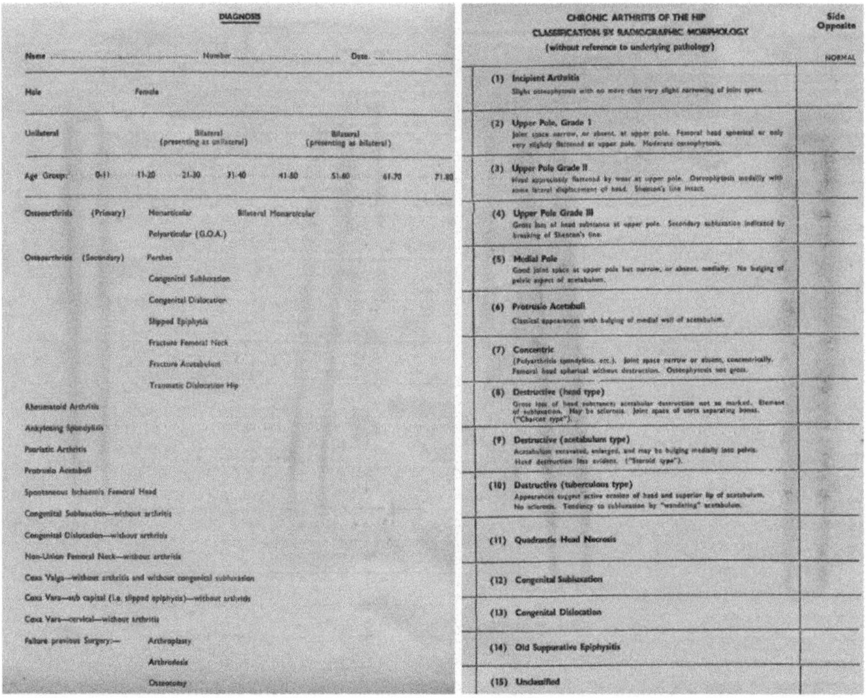

Fig. 6.1 Yellow radiographic assessment chart noting the underlying hip pathology and the radiographic appearance of the arthritic hip

Radiographic Morphology of the Arthritic Hip [1]

Uniformity of terminology and agreement on definitions are an essential part of scientific communication. It allows meaningful comparisons, avoids anecdotal presentations or emotional overtones and contributes to the advancement of our knowledge. In the arthritic hip, where radiographic appearances usually change with time, a statement: "severe arthritis" or "end stage arthritis" – has no meaning; it probably reflects the surgeon's or the patient's emotions more accurately.

Drawing lines or diagrams on hard-copy radiographs is best avoided, unless they can be easily removed without damaging the radiograph. Although they may serve a purpose, temporarily, they only attract the attention of the viewer; maybe to the exclusion of more important pathology. Eventually the reason for the lines is forgotten. The possibility of making errors when too much reliance is placed "on the lines drawn on radiographs …and used as a basis for calculation" has been pointed out [2]. With the computer technology used today the problem is no longer relevant.

Incipient Arthritis

Very slight narrowing of joint space. Although looked for superiorly it can be observed infero-medially. Subarticular sclerosis and a small inferior marginal acetabular osteophyte, running parallel with the joint line, may be present (Fig. 6.2).

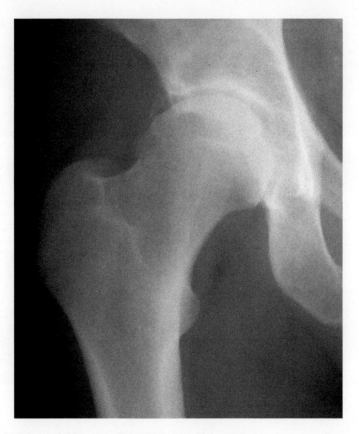

Fig. 6.2 Incipient arthritis – very slight narrowing of joint space

Upper Pole Grade I

Joint space narrow, or absent, at upper pole. Femoral head spherical or only very slightly flattened at the upper pole. Moderate osteophytes may be present.

Upper Pole Grade II

Head appreciably flattened at the upper pole. Medial acetabular osteophyte with some lateral displacement of the head.

Fig. 6.3 Upper pole grade II – head appreciably flattened at the upper pole. Medial acetabular osteophyte with some lateral displacement of the head

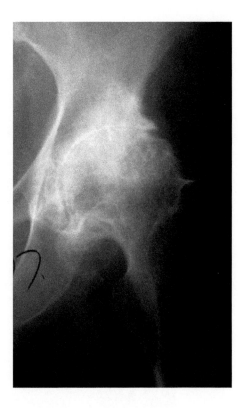

If Shenton's line is used to define normal anatomy then it can be expected to be intact in the three types of arthritis described above. It must be accepted that Shenton's line is probably more accurately defined as a band; the limits of normality lie within that band – it is not a single line (Fig. 6.3).

Upper Pole Grade III

Gross loss of head substance with flattening of the upper pole. Secondary subluxation with breaking of the Shenton's "line" (Fig. 6.4)

Medial Pole

Good joint space at the upper pole but becomes narrow, or even absent, medially. No bulging of the medial wall of the acetabulum (Fig. 6.5).

Protrusio Acetabuli

Classical appearances with bulging of the medial acetabular wall (Fig. 6.6). (Note the histology [3].).

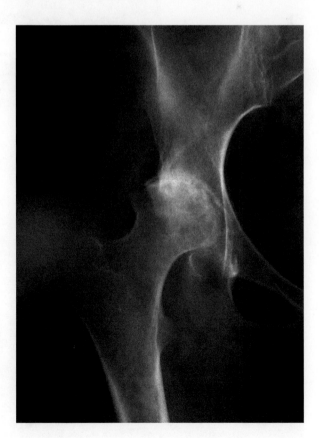

Fig. 6.4 Upper pole grade III gross loss of head substance with flattening of the upper pole

Fig. 6.5 Medial pole –
good joint space at the
upper pole but becomes
narrow, or even absent,
medially

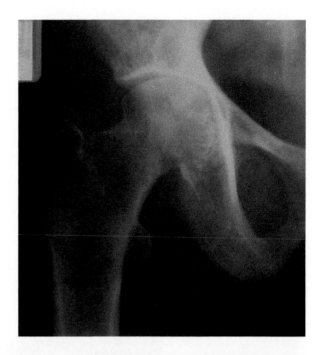

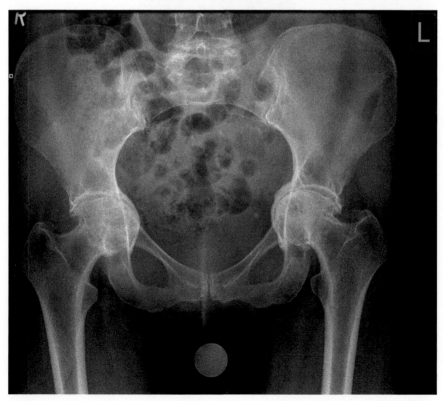

Fig. 6.6 Protrusio acetabuli – classical appearances with bulging of the medial acetabular wall

Concentric

Joint space narrowed or absent concentrically. Femoral head spherical without destruction. May indicate cartilage necrosis, inflammatory or early septic arthritis (Fig. 6.7).

Destructive

Involving mainly the femoral head or acetabulum or both. Rapid destruction of the femoral head within the acetabulum, relatively well preserved, especially in the early stages. May resemble neuropathic, Charcot type, with loss of bone substance – as if the bone was melting away. The destructive tuberculous type destroys the femoral head with bone remnants within the cavity and erosion of the superior lip of the acetabulum (Fig. 6.8).

Quadrantic Head Necrosis

The appearance will depend on the stage of presentation. Although with the advent of sophisticated investigations the diagnosis can be established earlier (Fig. 6.9).

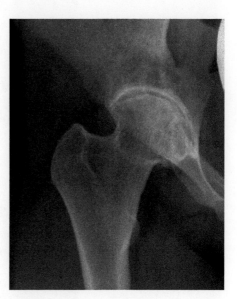

Fig. 6.7 Concentric – joint space narrowed or absent concentrically

Fig. 6.8 Destructive –
involving mainly the
femoral head or
acetabulum or both. Rapid
destruction of the femoral
head within the acetabulum

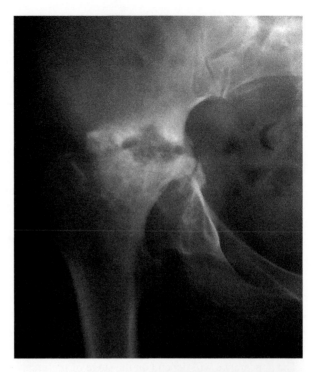

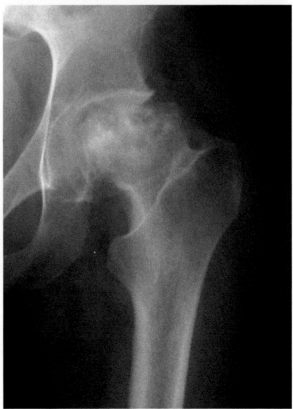

Fig. 6.9 Quadrantic head
necrosis – the appearance
will depend on the stage of
presentation

Fig. 6.10 Congenital
dysplasia, subluxation,
dislocation – a classical
appearance of a hip with
very variable radiographic
appearances: from no more
than a mildly sloping
acetabulum and deficient
femoral head cover to a
very small femoral head
approaching the iliac crest

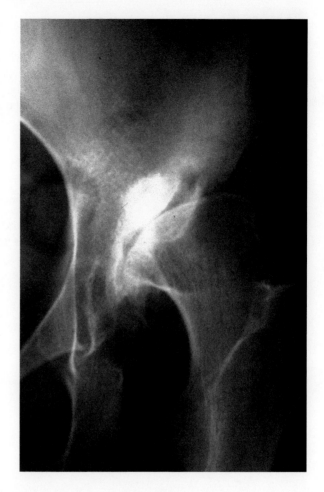

Congenital Dysplasia, Subluxation, Dislocation

A classical appearance of a hip with very variable radiographic appearances: from no more than a mildly sloping acetabulum and deficient femoral head cover to a very small femoral head approaching the iliac crest. Various classifications attempt to shade the severity of the condition by placing each one in a group. This may be interesting and even of help, but with such divergence of appearances, with merely an artificial division between grades, this is not an easy task (Fig. 6.10).

Unclassified

It is inevitable that in any classification there may be an unidentified group often bundled together as "other". In the context of hip pathology such a group need not be large for what we are attempting to describe is radiographic appearance and not to establish the true nature of the underlying pathology.

One other aspect must be mentioned. An instant success of total hip arthroplasty has, to a greater extent, eliminated the desire to study the understanding of underlying hip pathology in any detail or to consider other forms of treatment that may delay, even if not prevent, hip replacement at some future date. A sad loss to science.

The recent attention to mechanical aspects as "impingement syndrome" is a very welcome attempt to identify, intervene and possibly delay hip replacement.

References

1. Wroblewski BM, Charnley J. Radiographic morphology of the osteoarthritic hip. J Bone Joint Surg (Br). 1982;64-B:568–9.
2. Caterall RCF. Ex Umbris Erudito. J Bone Joint Surg (Br). 1968;50-B:455.
3. Wroblewski BM, Hillman F. Idiopathic protrusio acetabuli: a histological study. Clin Orthop Relat Res. 1979;138:228–30.

Chapter 7
Instrument Tray System

The surgical operation is divided into seven convenient stages and the instruments for each stage are kept permanently in separate trays

Tray system, as introduced by Charnley for his operation of hip replacement, or in fact any system which provides a sterile set of instruments and drapes for any invasive procedure, is now a standard practice. It must be appreciated, however, that until the tray system was adopted it was customary to have a collection of instruments laid out for the whole operating session, often lasting several hours! The table was covered with a sterile drape which was lifted as the instruments were taken or added to.

With the instrument tray system in place, the theatre, with its clean air unidirectional downward flow and the total body exhausts, virtually becomes an extension of the autoclave.

The tray system imposes discipline which ensures uninterrupted flow of the well rehearsed operation.

The Seven Tray System for the Charnley LFA

Each of the seven trays contained the instruments essential for the particular stage of the operation, but a number of these had clearly to be retained till a later or even the final stage of the procedure e.g. retractors or skin isolation towel clips.

Tray 1	Skin incision to deep fascia, haemostasis and isolation of cut skin edges with towels (Fig. 7.1)
Tray 2	Incision of deep fascia, initial incision retractor, trochanteric osteotomy using Gigli saw, dislocation of the hip and section of the femoral neck (Fig. 7.2)
Tray 3	Exposure and preparation of the acetabulum. Cementing of the acetabular cup (Fig. 7.3)

© Springer International Publishing Switzerland 2016
B.M. Wroblewski et al., *Charnley Low-Frictional Torque Arthroplasty of the Hip: Practice and Results*, DOI 10.1007/978-3-319-21320-0_7

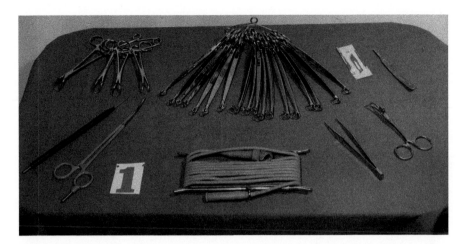

Fig. 7.1 Tray number 1. Skin incision to deep fascia, haemostasis and isolation of cut skin edges with towels

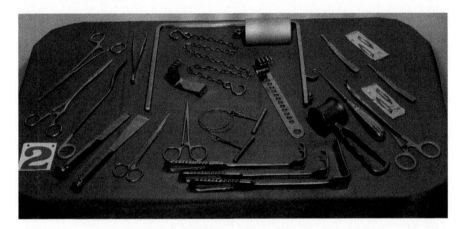

Fig. 7.2 Tray number 2. Incision of deep fascia, initial incision retractor, trochanteric osteotomy using Gigli saw, dislocation of the hip and section of the femoral neck

Tray 4	Exposure of the medullary canal, trial reduction, distal closure with bone block (Fig. 7.4)
Tray 5	Final preparation of the medullary canal, introduction of wires for trochanteric reattachment, cement injection and pressurisation, stem insertion (Fig. 7.5)
Tray 6	Reattachment of the greater trochanter (Fig. 7.6)
Tray 7	Wound closure in layers: the abductors with the reattached trochanter, deep fascia, fat and skin (Fig. 7.7)

The important aspect of the instrument tray system is the discipline that becomes the integral part of each stage of the operation. Thus, each stage must be completed in such a manner as to allow an uninterrupted and continuous progress for the

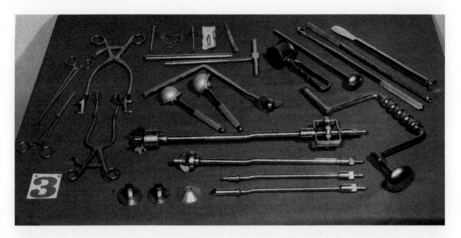

Fig. 7.3 Tray number 3. Exposure and preparation of the acetabulum. Cementing of the acetabular cup

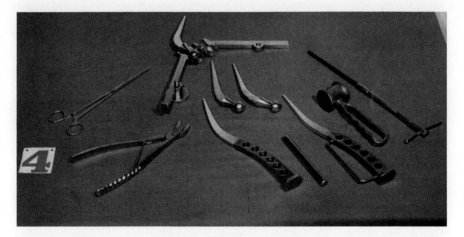

Fig. 7.4 Tray number 4. Exposure of the medullary canal, trial reduction, distal closure with bone block, introduction of wires for trochanteric reattachment

operation as a whole. What is not readily appreciated, is that the lack of progress during the operation is the most frustrating aspect that leads to loss of concentration, use of force and tissue damage. It is this lack of progress that makes any routine operation "a difficult operation". The staging of the operation and the use of the instrument tray system go a long way to avoid this. Experience has shown that with a routine LFA the number of trays can be reduced; the minimum depending on the surgeon's routine, skill and the support offered by the theatre staff. Operating time is for surgery and not for searching for instruments or prostheses or discussing the latest news item. A suggestion that a surgeon must have a wide selection of instruments for an elective procedure "in case they may be needed" cannot be correct. Elective surgery is about making the decision before the operation and maintaining an uninterrupted progress throughout the operation.

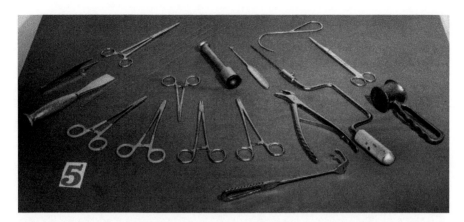

Fig. 7.5 Tray number 5. Final preparation of the medullary canal, cement injection and pressurisation, stem insertion

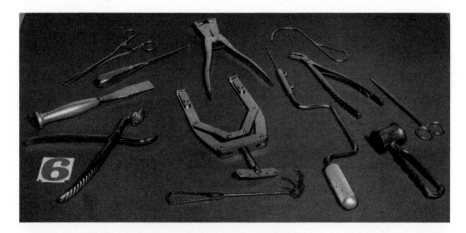

Fig. 7.6 Tray number 6. Reattachment of the greater trochanter

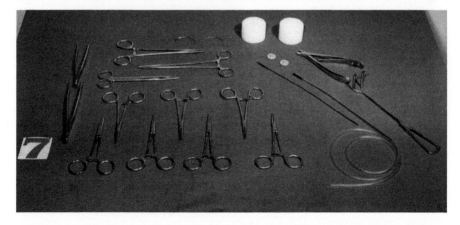

Fig. 7.7 Tray number 7. Wound closure in layers: the abductors with the reattached trochanter, deep fascia, fat and skin

Chapter 8
Exposure of the Hip Joint

If it could be guaranteed that the greater trochanter would unite within three weeks when reattached, and without imposing restrictions which would impede rehabilitation, few surgeons would fail to avail themselves of the easy and beautiful access to the hip joint provided by the approach (1979)

In the evolution of the LFA and its introduction into clinical practice Charnley pursued the ideal of mechanical perfection; trochanteric osteotomy and reattachment was part of that philosophy. Even when he was ready to put his final version of the technique of the LFA into print Charnley stated: *"Dissatisfaction with reattachment* (of the trochanter) *has been the cause of many years of delay in writing this book. A method which satisfies the author has at last been found"*.

Our objective is to present some aspects of the history and evolution of this method of exposure, show the results and leave it to others to comment, judge and decide by their own experience and long-term results, provided of course that these are continually reviewed.

Historical Aspect

It is probably correct to suggest, on Charnley's own admission, that it was the late Sir Harry Platt who introduced Charnley to this method of hip exposure. Whoever was the first to introduce this method into clinical practice, it was certainly not for the purpose of total hip arthroplasty. This was the only method that Charnley used routinely for his operation of the LFA. It was not merely for easy access and good exposure, Charnley followed the teaching of Pauwels. Any attempt of reducing the load on the hip joint must include balancing and improving the lever ratios; reducing the medial lever: from the centre of the rotation of the femoral head to mid-line of the body, while increasing the lateral lever: from the centre of the rotation to the lateral aspect of the greater trochanter [1] (Fig. 8.1). Trochanteric osteotomy lends itself to that concept.

© Springer International Publishing Switzerland 2016
B.M. Wroblewski et al., *Charnley Low-Frictional Torque Arthroplasty of the Hip: Practice and Results*, DOI 10.1007/978-3-319-21320-0_8

Fig. 8.1 Reducing the load on the hip joint must include balancing and improving the lever ratios; reducing the medial lever: from the centre of the rotation of the femoral head to mid-line of the body, while increasing the lateral lever: from the centre of the rotation to the lateral aspect of the greater trochanter

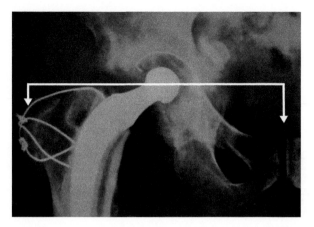

The Cup

The cup was medialised by reaming the acetabulum, while the trochanter was placed laterally and distally. There was nothing wrong with the concept: what came later sheds some light on the subject. In the original description of the operative technique, the perforator, the deepening and expanding reamers, were all directed towards the patient's opposite shoulder. The depth was judged by the thickness of the acetabular floor remaining after reaming, thus medialising the cup. To indicate the advantages of lateral and distal placement of the greater trochanter numerical values were used: position 3 – trochanter placed on its original bed; position 1 – trochanter reattached distally past its bed onto the lateral aspect of the shaft of the femur; position 2 – intermediate between 1 and 3 (Fig. 8.2).

Was the theoretical benefit of medialisation of the cup reflected in the long-term results? Did medialised cups wear less when compared with the rim supported cup? Availability of long term results offered the information (refer to Wear chapter).

The Stem

The medullary canal was approached through the sectioned neck, the trochanteric bed was not encroached upon and as a result the stem was often in a varus position. The intact trochanteric cancellous bed offered a large area of contact, the leg was not lengthened and the patient stayed in bed for up to 3 weeks.

The Trochanter

The method of trochanteric osteotomy, reattachment and the excellent exposure did not attract attention: there were no problems! At this stage of evolution of the operation visiting surgeons admired Charnley's skill, the excellent exposure offered by

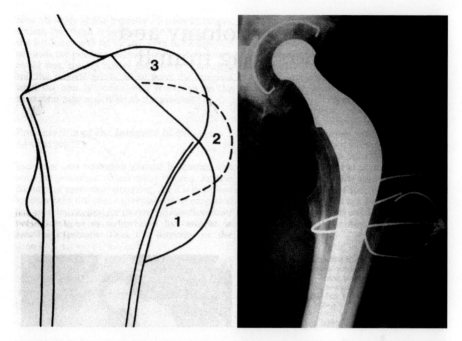

Fig. 8.2 Radiograph and diagram showing the advantages of lateral and distal placement of the greater trochanter: position *3* – trochanter placed on its original bed; position *1* – trochanter reattached distally past its bed onto the lateral aspect of the shaft of the femur; position *2* – in between 1 and 3 (Reproduced from: Wroblewski [6]. First described by Charnley [7])

trochanteric osteotomy and above all the ease of preparation of the medullary canal and cementing of the stem. Visitors were impressed: perforation of the femoral cortex, let alone the periprosthetic fractures, using the exposure, did not occur.

Post-Operative Routine

"The average stay in hospital is eight weeks" (1961). The post-operative management had clearly a role to play. *"After the earlier operations a single plaster hip spica was applied but in the last two years it has been found unnecessary to use anything more than a special triangular pillow between the knees."* (The reason for this apparently sudden change was that one patient – while awaiting application of the plaster – fell out of bed. No damage was done, henceforth, no plaster spica). *"Full weight bearing is permitted at 3 weeks"* (1963).

Changing Patterns

This digression to the very origins of the LFA technique must not be seen to be out of place. Surgery of the hip joint was evolving. Tuberculosis was the common problem. Improvements in sanitation, screening and vaccination resulted in the decline of the disease. Advent of anti-tuberculous drugs allowed surgical intervention and early mobilisation reducing the length of inpatient stay from years to months or even weeks.

Attention was now focused on the arthritic hip. Hip fusion, osteotomy and plaster fixation, then internal fixation and early mobilisation was merely a changing pattern of hip pathology presenting for the available treatment. Eight weeks of bed rest after the LFA was, by comparison, a tremendous advance. Even the most recent changes allowing discharge within days of surgery must be viewed as the changing pattern imposed by changing indications, type of surgery, patient selection, availability of after-care facilities, as well as the financial implications of medical treatment in general and not some newly discovered principle.

Changing Practice

A number of events coming in quick succession changed the practice. In an attempt to reduce the already very low post-operative dislocation rate, transverse reaming of the acetabulum was advocated, bringing the cup down to the anatomical level. The first fractured stem presented in 1968. While this complication was still in single figures it was clear that the stem was often in varus position; valgus and even excessive valgus became the teaching. What followed was more obvious, in retrospect. Transverse reaming of the acetabulum and anatomical position of the cup lengthened the limb. The stem, now in valgus, not only lengthened the limb further but also encroached into the cancellous bed of the trochanter. The trochanter would not come to lie "peacefully" onto its bed now with a reduced area of contact; it had to be reattached with the hip in an abduction position. The patients were encouraged to get up early: "Pillow for 5 days, up at 2 days" – became the post-operative routine: The result: trochanteric non-union.

The explanation – a pain free mobile hip allows free adduction movement, this may lift the trochanter off its bed slackening the wires which then fail by fatigue and also in a brittle manner. It was during this period that numerous methods of trochanteric reattachment were designed and tested both experimentally and clinically. It is this sequence of events that became the source of polarization of opinions on the exposure.

Some surgeons, observing Charnley at surgery during this period, looked askance and with scepticism as Charnley's hands moved swiftly both taking off and reattaching the trochanter. Some even considered it to be Charnley's "fly paper" or a "mousetrap"!

When Charnley brought in his Neck Length Jig, and the latest method of trochanteric reattachment: *"the problem of the trochanter has been truly solved,"* adding what appeared to be yet a further complexity to the operation, the pattern was set – for or against trochanteric osteotomy. Yet Charnley was aiming, once again, for mechanical perfection: central position of the stem within the medullary canal, correct leg length and therefore stability of the joint and secure reattachment of the trochanter.

As a result of these events a number of exposures of the hip joint were described, most of them based on the original Mcfarland-Osborne, (1984) the Liverpool, approach. The McFarland and Osborne exposure of the hip joint was based on that of Kocher (1909). McFarland and Osborne stated that their exposure "… depends on the anatomical observation that the gluteus medius and vastus lateralis <u>can be regarded as being in direct functional continuity</u> through the thick "tendinous" periosteum covering the greater trochanter" [2]. A number of authors in their modifications of this exposure misquote the original by stating that the two muscles <u>are</u> in functional continuity. They also fail to take into account both the anatomy and the function of the two muscles by disregarding the important statement made in the original: "… these two muscles meet at an angle, open anteriorly, so that by loosening the periosteum from the trochanter it is possible to displace forward the combined muscle fibres like bucket handle."

Fascial continuity between the gluteus medius and vastus lateralis is a fact, functional continuity is not: gluteus medius acts across the hip joint, vastus lateralis across the knee and there is no sling between the two for example as in external oblique of the eye. Gluteus medius arises from the outer surface of the ilium and also from gluteal aponeurosis covering its outer surface. The fibres converge to a strong flattened tendon which is inserted into the oblique line on the outer surface of the greater trochanter.

When viewed from the lateral aspect at the exposure of the hip, two distinctive parts of the gluteus medius are clearly seen. The bulk of the muscle belly runs from the pelvis to the antero-lateral part of the greater trochanter and forms a right angle with the shaft of the femur. The lesser part of the muscle fibres run in line with the long axis of the femur (Fig. 8.3).

This angle between the bulk of the gluteus medius and the greater trochanter becomes ever more acute as the head of the femur migrates proximally; it is most obvious in congenital dislocation of the hip.

Although the muscle is fan-shaped it is not symmetrical with respect to the greater trochanter and the femoral shaft – bulk of it lies anteriorly. This anatomy has

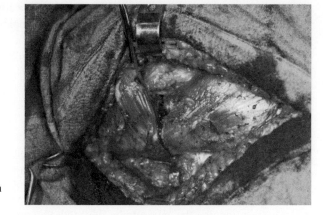

Fig. 8.3 Exposure at operation. Loss of this anterior part of the muscle leads to loss of active internal rotation of the hip and can be spotted early on clinical examination

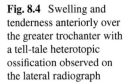

Fig. 8.4 Swelling and tenderness anteriorly over the greater trochanter with a tell-tale heterotopic ossification observed on the lateral radiograph

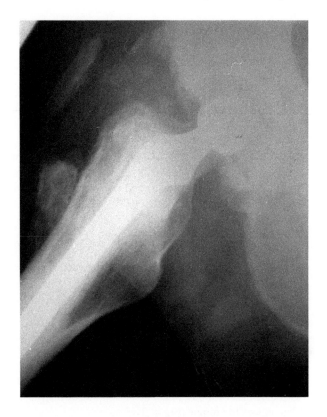

clear functional implications. The main function is that of a flexor – internal rotator of the hip (a number of publications, with line drawings of gluteus medius, are incorrect; they show the muscle as a symmetrically placed fan arrangement of a pure abductor). Loss of this anterior part of the muscle leads to loss of active internal rotation of the hip and can be spotted early on clinical examination. With the loss of the anterior part of the gluteus medius, what is left of the muscle, are the vertical fibres which merely act as a 'bucket handle' not controlling external rotation. The result of this complication may present clinically as a swelling and tenderness anteriorly over the greater trochanter with a tell-tale heterotopic ossification observed on the lateral radiograph (Fig. 8.4).

It is here that most misunderstandings of the function and the role of the gluteous medius in total hip replacement arise.

Trochanteric Osteotomy

In a speciality as vast as that of orthopaedics surgeons yearn for an easy hip operation. (1960)

Trochanteric osteotomy appears to make the operation more complex because it brings yet a further demand – the reattachment of the trochanter. There are no publications condemning the exposure by this method – objections if any, can only be levelled at the need and method of reattachment and any complications arising. (It is interesting to note that "an extended trochanteric osteotomy" or even splitting of the femur has found favour with surgeons who have hitherto avoided trochanteric osteotomy. It is probably correct to point out that cerclage wire, placed around the shaft of the femur, opened at revision, has become acceptable: the advocates of this method are probably more familiar with this part of the anatomy.

Any arguments for or against the osteotomy should not become a major issue if it is clearly understood what is required at surgery and what are the mechanical objectives for which the operation was designed. This bone of contention should be put to rest. Revisions will clearly demand that the issue be revisited by those not familiar with this method of exposure.

Aims of Exposure

Circumferential view of the acetabulum and direct access to the medullary canal and not through the neck of the femur. (An intramedullary nail enters through the piriformis fossa – not through the femoral neck) (Fig. 8.5).

In the earliest publication on the subject of trochanteric osteotomy in arthroplasty of the hip Charnley and Ferriera [1] outlined the reasons for, the method of osteotomy, the reattachment, as well as the results including the union rate. The overall union rate was 92.9 %. The most distal and lateral transposition of the trochanter had the highest union rate: 97.4 % as well as the greatest improvement in the post-operative range of abduction of the hip.

Slip of the greater trochanter from its original position was observed in 19.6 % of cases but most of these, 81.8 %, proceeded to union. Some comments on this study may not be out of place in order to highlight some aspects of this part of the procedure. Measuring the active range of movements of an arthritic joint in order to test the integrity of a group of muscles, can only be valid if a passive range of movement is possible. The highest union rate (97.4 %) with the most distal placement of the greater trochanter (POSITION ONE) is rather unexpected as compared with the highest failure rate of 10.8 % with the greater trochanter returning to its original place (POSITION THREE).

What is not usually appreciated, and is documented in the publication, is that a slip of the trochanter after its reattachment may occur, (19.6 % in this series) with most of them, 36 of 34 (81.8 %) resulting in union.

Biplanar Trochanteric Osteotomy

The biplaner trochanteric osteotomy was based on the original suggestion made by Debeyre and Duliveux [3] and the subsequent description by Weber and Stuhmer [4]. This method had the advantage of increasing the area in contact of the greater

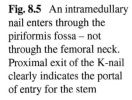

Fig. 8.5 An intramedullary
nail enters through the
piriformis fossa – not
through the femoral neck.
Proximal exit of the K-nail
clearly indicates the portal
of entry for the stem

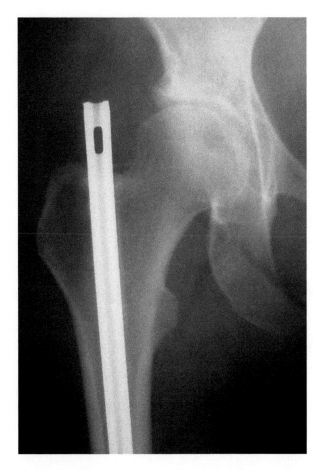

trochanter with the bony bed and also resisting rotation once in contact. The oscillating saw was used to achieve the biplanar shape.

   The disadvantage of using an oscillating saw is the ease with which the trochanter could be overcut over its summit, plus the fact that the osteotomy is extracapsu-
lar. The biplanar osteotomy, when cut with a Gigli saw, is intracapsular and,
therefore, facilitates dislocation of the hip. The method and results have been
described [5] (Figs. 8.6 and 8.7).

   In a prospective study the results of biplanar trochanteric osteotomy and the three
methods of re-attachment were tested [5] (Table 8.1).

Note The higher number of revisions and previous hip operations in the double
wire and compression spring group reflect the clinical practice. It was an interesting
observation that with this method of trochanteric reattachment there were no cases
of fractured wires <u>and</u> bony union.

Discussion

The question must remain: what is the role of trochanteric osteotomy in the attempts to improve lever ratios, to medialise the centre of rotation of the hip or lateralise the greater trochanter? After all this was one of the explanations proposed by Charnley. The answer is: probably very little – but for different, practical reasons. The concept of improving lever ratios remains valid, as is the need for full exposure for the purpose of sound fixation of the components. What has changed is the clinical practice.

The restoration, and even improvement, of the lever ratios can be achieved by careful pre-operative planning, full exposure at surgery and the selection of appropriate components and their correct placement.

Trochanteric osteotomy now becomes a method of exposure to achieve the planned objectives. It is the technical developments made possible by the accumulation of information and selection of sizes of cups, but above all, of stems with variable offsets and neck lengths that made it possible to achieve the same objective by a different route.

Choice of range of stem offsets, neck lengths and possibly of various levels of modular head seating may appear to be an advantage because adjustments can be carried out during the operation. Careful pre-operative planning reduces the need

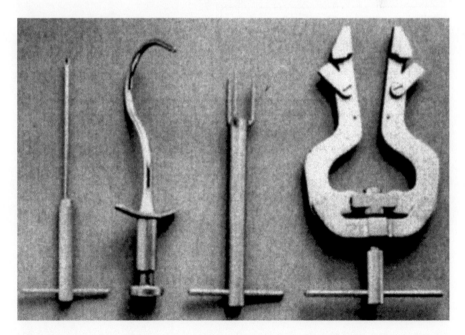

Fig. 8.6 Trochanteric spike, wire passer, tident for positioning the trochanteric fragment and wire tightener

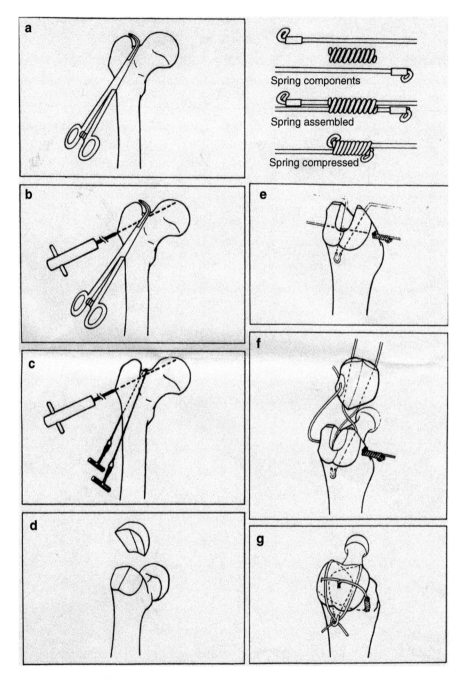

Spring components

Spring assembled

Spring compressed

Fig. 8.7 The technique of biplanar intracapsular trochanteric osteotomy with method of re-attachment. The biplanar osteotomy, when cut with a Gigli saw is intracapsular and therefore facilitates dislocation of the hip. (Reproduced with permission and copyright of the British Editorial Society of Bone and Joint Surgery from Wroblewski and Shelley [5])

Table 8.1 Biplanar trochanteric osteotomy, methods of fixation and radiographic results

Method of reattachment	Primary LFA	Previous hip operations	Revisions of Failed THA	Non-union	
				No	(%)
Cruciate wire	45	14	7	5	(7.6)
Double and single wire	94	27	18	11	(7.9)
Double wire and compression spring	77	35	114	4	(1.8)

for availability of a "selection of implants" during the operation. Availability of variations, without pre-operative planning, may put off the decision time till the very last moment, when the required variation may not be forthcoming; or becomes merely the only unavoidable, but not necessarily the optimal, option.

Surgeons planning to become seriously involved in total hip arthroplasty will eventually have to face their own, and possibly colleagues' cases, for revision surgery. It can be argued that this is the wrong time to start adding another procedure, trochanteric osteotomy, be it standard or extended, and its reattachment, to what may not be an easy revision. Single case satisfaction remains the driving force of clinical practice. The ultimate benefit of revision lies in the information gained to improve primary procedures. The challenge of ever more complex revisions must not overshadow the fact that most long-term benefits will come from well carried out primary procedures. In this context the exposure of the hip by trochanteric osteotomy is yet to be improved upon.

References

1. Charnley J, de Ferreira SD. Transplantation of the greater trochanter in arthroplasty of the hip. J Bone Joint Surg (Br). 1964;46B:191–7.
2. McFarland B, Osborne G. Approach to the hip: a suggested improvement on Kocher's method. J Bone Joint Surg. 1954;36B:364–7.
3. Debeyre Y, Duliveux P. Les arthroplasties de la hanche; etude critique a propos de 200 cas operes. Paris: Editous Medicales Flammarion; 1954.
4. Weber BG, Stuhmer G. Improvements in total hip prosthesis implantation technique: a cement-proof seal for the lower medullary cavity and a dihedral self-stabilising trochanteric osteotomy. Arch Orthop Trauma Surg. 1979;93(3):185–9.
5. Wroblewski BM, Shelley P. Reattachment of the greater trochanter after hip replacement. J Bone Joint Surg (Br). 1985;67B:736–40.
6. Wroblewski BM. Revision surgery in total hip arthroplasty. London: Springer; 1990.
7. Charnley J. Total prosthetic replacement for advanced coxarthrosis. Sicot X Congress, Paris; 1966. p. 316.

Chapter 9
Post-operative Length of Hospital Stay

The patient is splinted with the leg in abduction for three weeks, and is allowed to take full weight on the hip five weeks after the operation. Recent experiences suggest that the plaster is not essential. The average stay in hospital is eight weeks. Charnley 1961

To a newcomer to the surgery of total hip arthroplasty the statement may appear to be like something from the very early days of surgery; in fact it was – from the very early days of total hip arthroplasty.

It may be, even if only of historical interest, to revisit the past of both Wrightington Hospital and the Centre for Hip Surgery.

The Hospital became functional in early 1932 with the official opening on 16th June 1932 (Fig. 9.1). By that date over 300 visitors have signed the visitors book – amongst them Sir Robert Jones on 2nd October 1932 (Fig. 9.2).

The location was selected, so that the Hospital, when built, would serve as a "refuge" for patients, primarily children with tuberculosis, away from the pollution of the industrial revolution. The treatment available was: rest, fresh air and good food, with some sessions of artificial light. Visiting surgeons from surrounding cities carried out outpatient and operating sessions. The treatment of bone and joint tuberculosis and correction of deformities included prolonged uninterrupted rest, to give nature the time to heal. Immobilisation in the plaster of Paris (p-o-p) either individual joints or more extensive parts with p-o-p spica or plaster bed was the method. The length of inpatient stay was measured in months and even years. Children with Perthes disease of the hip were, at times, included in this mode of treatment. The availability of anti-tuberculous drugs changed all that – it allowed early surgery and mobilisation. Combined with improved sanitation, nutrition and inoculation, TB was no longer the problem it has been. Hospital beds became available.

Osteoarthritis of the major joints, the hip and the knee, came to the forefront. Corrective osteotomy and joint fusion with p-o-p immobilisation shortened the length of inpatient stay from years to months. Internal fixation, then compression fixation, obviated the need for external immobilisation, allowed early mobilisation

© Springer International Publishing Switzerland 2016

B.M. Wroblewski et al., *Charnley Low-Frictional Torque Arthroplasty of the Hip: Practice and Results*, DOI 10.1007/978-3-319-21320-0_9

Opening Day Programme

COUNTY COUNCIL.

Formal Opening

OF THE

Wrightington Hospital

near Wigan,

ON

16th June (Friday), 1933,

BY

Sir GEORGE NEWMAN, K.C.B., M.D.,
F.R.C.P., Hon. D.C.L., LL.D., F.R.C.S.

Chief Medical Officer of the Ministry of Health.

---

p.m.   PROGRAMME.

2-45   Assembly of guests at the Wrightington Hospital and recep-
to   tion by County Alderman J. T. Travis-Clegg, D.L., J.P.,
2-55   Chairman of the Lancashire County Council, who will take the
           chair.

3-0   Introductory remarks by the Chairman, who on conclusion will
           call on Sir George Newman to open the door (the key to be pre-
           sented by Col. C. J. Trimble) and to address the assembly.   Sir
           George Newman, after opening the door and declaring the
           Hospital officially open, will return to the platform and deliver
           an address.

           Vote of thanks to Sir George Newman.

              Proposer : Col. C. J. Trimble, C.B., C.M.G., Chairman of the
                   County Tuberculosis Committee.

              Seconder : County Alderman J. C. Beckitt, M.R.C.S., L.R.C.P.,
                   D.P.H.

           Reply by Sir George Newman.

           Vote of thanks to the Chairman.

              Proposer : County Councillor E. Boothman, J.P., Vice-Chair-
                   man of the County Tuberculosis Committee.

           Reply by the Chairman.

                 GOD SAVE THE KING.

           Inspection of the Hospital and Grounds independently by the
           guests.

4-0 to 4-30.   Tea in marquee.

              (*For transport arrangements see page 8*).

Fig. 9.1 Official opening day programme of Wrightington Hospital 1932

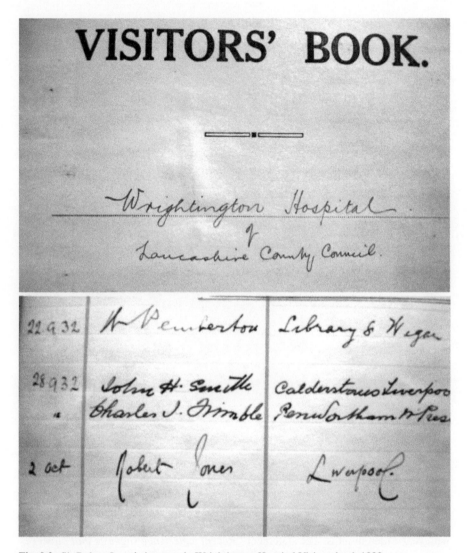

Fig. 9.2 Sir Robert Jones' signature in Wrightington Hospital Visitors book 1932

and discharge. It was at that stage that Charnley set out to investigate the possibility of total hip arthroplasty.

Originally the Centre for Hip Surgery was planned as a facility, not only for training surgeons, but also to investigate which method would be most suitable for patients with hip osteoarthritis. Four methods were considered: corrective osteotomy, fusion, excision or hip arthroplasty. Clearly arthroplasty was the most attractive method: *"because this is a reconstruction of a normal joint"* The planned role for the Centre for Hip Surgery was changing: with priority being – *"polyarthritis of the rheumatoid type, geriatric problems of painful hips and salvage of failures of previous operations on the hip."*

Fig. 9.3 Hip registers
from Wrightington
Hospital 1959, 1960, 1961

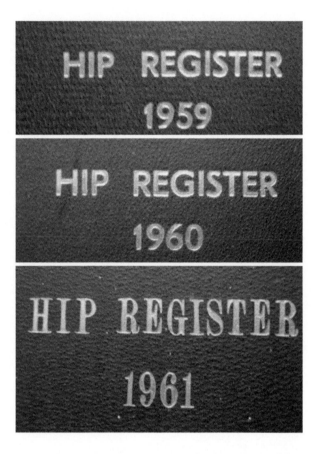

The Hip Register – established by Charnley in 1959 (Fig. 9.3) is a detailed record of every operation carried out during the 3 year period 1959–1961 with additional comments and observations.

With attempts at total hip arthroplasty the caution and delay in mobilisation was justified and the length of stay of 8 week does not seem excessive when compared with years, then months. The statement *"Recent experience suggests that plaster is not essential"* reveals the fact that patients were immobilised in p-o-p spica for up to 6 weeks and the *"recent experience"* was a patient that fell out of bed without any ill effect. With time, increasing confidence, at both ends of the scalpel, extension of health care away from the hospitals, as well as the pressures to reduce inpatient costs, the hospital bed is becoming merely an item on the "patient care pathway". The objective is for the patient to move through the system as fast as possible, while collecting as many or as few, depending on who is footing the bill, chargeable items, not unlike a visit to a supermarket.

It is not the objective to discuss merits or otherwise of any particular system but merely to offer some insight how the present practice is but a stage in the evolution of a continuing process.

One aspect must remain in the very forefront – the care given to the patient while an inpatient, and aftercare for the "lifetime of the arthroplasty" are the mandatory aspects of the treatment.

Chapter 10
Results of Low-Friction Arthroplasty of the Hip Performed as a Primary Intervention

"The clinical material relates to the hips operated on from November 1962, when high density polyethylene replaced Teflon for the acetabular component, to December 1965."
"Any attempt to compare the state of the hip before and after operation by use of numbers has obvious limitations." 1972.

Charnley's first publication on the results of the operation demands detailed study. It puts down foundations to so much of the subsequent work on the subject. The detailed clinical assessment, surgical technique, the post-operative care, complications and the results were documented. Uniformity of meaningful terminology is an essential part of scientific communication. Any attempt at pre-operative clinical assessment and documenting the results of surgery must be simple enough to collect and yet detailed to convey the essential information. Whatever the method used there will always be scope for improvement and modification, and above all for the need of "reading between the lines".

Surgical Technique

"The essential mechanical details of the technique employed in this series" – size of the head, the shape and size of the neck – were established from experience with Teflon. *"… Neutral anteversion (of the cup) is advised, with a maximum of 5 degrees of anteversion… The axis of the femoral prosthesis is neutral."* *"Both components are fixed with self-curing acrylic cement"*.

"Emphasis is laid on deepening the acetabulum until no more than two or three millimetres of bone is left in the floor." This was to medialise the cup, thus reducing the medial lever and improving the mechanical advantage by reducing the load on the hip – while the trochanter is transferred laterally and distally. (Did this technique produce expected results?)

© Springer International Publishing Switzerland 2016
B.M. Wroblewski et al., *Charnley Low-Frictional Torque Arthroplasty of the Hip: Practice and Results*, DOI 10.1007/978-3-319-21320-0_10

Post-operative Rehabilitation

Post-operative rehabilitation was conducted more slowly in this series – patients being confined to bed for up to 3 weeks with legs separated by an abduction pillow.

Results

Clinical (Fig. 10.1)

Charnley adopted the grading method of d'Aubigne and Postel (1954) [1] with modifications [2] to record pain, function and movement in the hip both pre-operatively and at follow-up. The description of this grading is noted in the clinical assessment section of the book.

Relief of pain The average grade for pain, before surgery, was 2.7 Average post-operative grading was 5.9.

Activity level for Grade A patients improved from 2.5 to 4.8.

Range of movements Although varying greatly between patients and the underlying hip pathology; the increase averaged from 2.7 to 5.2.

Dislocation

There were 9 early dislocations in the series of 582 arthroplasties (1.5 %). All were treated by closed reduction and non re-dislocated. There were no revisions for dislocation.

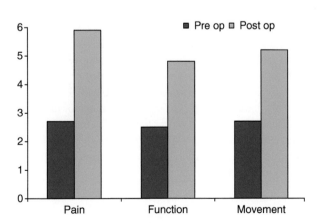

Fig. 10.1 Graph of clinical results – pain, function, movement. 1962–1965

Infection

Infection rate was 3.8 % of which 2.2 % were defined as "late".

Wear

Wear of the cup has shown considerable variations from 1 mm in 5 years to 0 at 7 years. Examination of explanted cups established the average penetration as 0.13 mm per year.

Charnley clearly appreciated the need for long-term follow-up: the minimum follow-up was 4 years (range 4–7 years), complications within the first year were included.

So what were the conclusions derived from this review of the 4–7 year results?

– As regards to pain relief and ability to walk, the average final rating was 90 % excellent and 10 % good.
– The average recovery of movement was influenced by the pre-operative range; it was improved though not spectacularly.
– There was no tendency to lose movement with the passage of time.
– When the socket was cemented the late mechanical failure from all causes was 1.3 % in 210 cases.
– The failure rate, excluding infection, was 3.8 %.

Comments

The question of histology of the bone cement interface in relation to any wear products would clearly have to await post-mortem specimens. In the context of assessment of functional results after hip replacement, popular press and commercial involvement, must also be mentioned. Single case patient satisfaction, can be visually demonstrated far better than a level of pain relief; it has a greater and longer lasting effect on the observer, hence the proliferation of advertising images. There is, however, a very important aspect of the practice of "single case success," anecdotal presentation; it is misleading.

Patient's activity level, after total hip arthroplasty, is not a characteristic of a particular design, nor of a method of component fixation, provided it is relatively secure under load: it is a reflection of patient selection for the operation.

These are invariably category **A** patients whose activity level was only temporarily restricted, and whose general condition allowed them to return to a high, even if only an early and temporary, level of activity. It is too obvious to point out that patients with multiple problems never feature as anecdotal single case successes.

The drawback of single case success is in the fact that it attracts patients with a high level of expectation of early benefit and has little understanding of the long-term commitment demanded by this form of treatment.

References

1. d'Aubigne RM, Postel M. Functional results of hip arthroplasty with acrylic prosthesis. J Bone Joint Surg (Am). 1954;36-A:451–75.
2. Charnley J. The long term results of low-friction arthroplasty of the hip as a primary intervention. J Bone Joint Surg (Br). 1972;84-B:61–76.

Chapter 11
Loosening of Components

Since absolute rigidity does not exist in nature, fixation of components and, therefore, failure of that fixation – loosening – may not be possible to define in terms that are acceptable to all.

In order to understand the complexity and the clinical significance of component loosening in total hip arthroplasty, it may be of interest to consider two aspects of this method of treatment: the indications for the operation and the reasons for clinical success.

The indications are brought on by the mechanical breakdown of the articulation. The clinical presentation is hip pain [1] restriction of movement of the joint and the activity of the patient.

Clinical success in correctly selected patients, is primarily due to pain relief as a result of the operation; the natural symptomatic articulation is replaced with an artificial neuropathic spacer functioning within a foreign body bursa.

Activity level achieved as a result of the operation is not a feature of a particular type of arthroplasty; it is a reflection of patient selection. Patents with multiple disabilities never feature as anecdotal single case successes.

The operation imposes demands on the technical skills of the surgeon: exposure of the joint, preparation of the bony bed and fixation of the components. Component fixation and their loosening may, therefore, be thought of as a "by-product" of this method of treatment.

The implant, now functioning as part of the skeleton, alters the patterns of load transfer with strain shielding and strain concentration. This gradual process is asymptomatic.

Failure of component fixation – loosening is an unknown experience to the patient and the surgeon. It is commonly and erroneously assumed that clinical success indicates secure component fixation and that failure of fixation will become clinically symptomatic. (A quotation on the subject, recorded during one of the past orthopaedic meetings, may be of interest. "If it did not trouble the patient it could not be a problem to the surgeon" shows the lack of understanding of the problem). Being a process its onset may not be obvious, nor may it be continuous or uniformly progressive.

© Springer International Publishing Switzerland 2016   93
B.M. Wroblewski et al., *Charnley Low-Frictional Torque Arthroplasty of the Hip:
Practice and Results*, DOI 10.1007/978-3-319-21320-0_11

Progressive loosening leads to failures of the skeleton housing the implant. Such failures present late, are symptomatic, possibly sudden in onset and result in loss of bone stock or fracture! Having reached that stage, the original problem, which was basically restricted to the articulating surfaces, now becomes a problem involving the skeleton. The technical problems to be addressed are now more in keeping with trauma and tumour surgery and not merely with the failure of the articulation.

To understand these features of both the natural joint and the arthroplasty, is to appreciate that clinical results do not reflect the mechanical state of the arthroplasty. Good quality serial radiographs offer more valuable information. The consequences of this method of surgery must be understood and accepted by the surgeon, the patient, and the health service **before** the operation.

Radiographic Appearances and Clinical Results

Clinical practice is driven largely by symptomatic patients. Having established the diagnosis, instituted appropriate treatment and relieved the symptoms, it is assumed that the problem has been solved. Any further problems would be expected to present symptomatically. This is the teaching, training and our practice. Prevention, anticipation and early intervention lag very far behind.

It should come as no surprise that the same reasoning is often applied to total hip arthroplasty as a method of treatment for painful, arthritic hips.

The Correlation Between Radiographic Appearances and Clinical Results

The correlation between the radiographic appearance of the cup and the findings at revision has been established by Hodgkinson et al. [2]. It was, therefore, logical that the study should be extended further in order to examine the correlation between radiographic appearances of the arthroplasty and the clinical results. Could we rely on patient's symptoms when anticipating mechanical problems after THA?

A group of 261 patients (320 LFAs) and their radiographs were reviewed at a mean follow up of 22 years and 10 months (20–30 years). Of these, 93.9 % were considered to be clinically successful; 82.3 % were free from pain and 11.6 % had no more than occasional discomfort. Function was satisfactory in 59.6 % and 62 % had an excellent range of movement [3] (A more detailed analysis of the results is shown in Table 11.1).

For the purpose of this study the radiological loosening of the cup was defined as change in position of the cup as observed on serial radiographs. Failure of stem fixation was classed according to Harris et al. [4] into "definite", "probable or "possible".

Clinical results did not correlate well with the radiographic appearances. Radiologically loose components did not affect the clinical results to the extent as to distinguish them from the radiologically secure ones. Even in the extreme cases where both components were radiologically secure or radiologically loose, the difference for pain relief was only 0.9 of a point and therefore classed as a clinically successful result.

Table 11.1 Correlation between radiographic appearances and clinical results

Radiological appearances	% Patients	Clinical outcome Charnley scores (average)		
		Pain	Function	Movement
Loose cup and stem	2.9	5.0	4.0	4.5
Loose cup secure stem	15.5	5.5	4.3	4.6
Secure cup loose stem	10.8	5.6	4.3	4.5
Secure cup and stem	70.8	5.8	4.9	4.8

Fig. 11.1 Charnley
press-fit cup. The implant,
radiograph
post-operatively

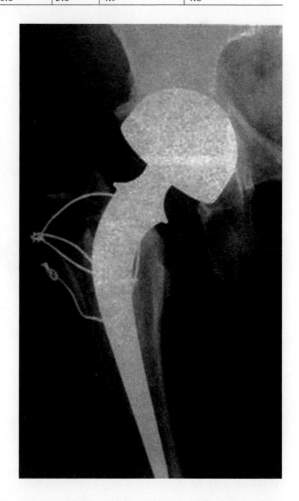

The commonest cause of long-term failures, cup loosening, could not be anticipated if reliance was placed purely on patients' symptoms. This should not come as
a surprise: the original Charnley (metal-backed) press-fit cups have never been
fixed. They were intended to spin on the spigot, by design, and thus avoid a unidirectional wear path. They were clinically successful; the longest follow-up (40 years)
was of that particular design (Figs. 11.1 and 11.2). The fact that the design was
given up was because of the high incidence of tilting and dislocation. With this
information in mind it becomes clear that any method of cup "fixation" can be

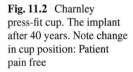

Fig. 11.2 Charnley
press-fit cup. The implant
after 40 years. Note change
in cup position: Patient
pain free

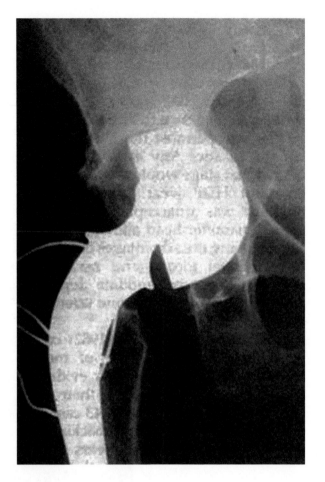

claimed to be successful clinically. It is the radiographic changes, occurring with time, that will determine the mechanical outcome. To study this aspect with good quality radiographs is essential.

Why should loose cups in THA remain asymptomatic? It could be argued that the acetabular side of the articulation is "less sensitive." (Hemi-arthroplasties, as used for fractures of the neck of the femur and avascular necrosis, were asymptomatic until the metal head bored into the acetabular floor). In total hip arthroplasty, the situation may be different. A cup, which is loose, will have a tendency to move when under load. Because of the sphericity of the cup and an eccentricity of the load, a closed system between the implant and the acetabulum cannot result: any part of the cup under compression will also result in a tilt of the cup and a release of pressure as the cup tilts away from the acetabular floor. This is supported by the lack of finding of localised cavitation at the bone-cement interface unless around a cement peg (Figs. 11.3 and 11.4) (It is only when a well fixed cup has reached the stage of complete wear-out, and fracture of the shell remnant, that it will present symptomatically) [5].

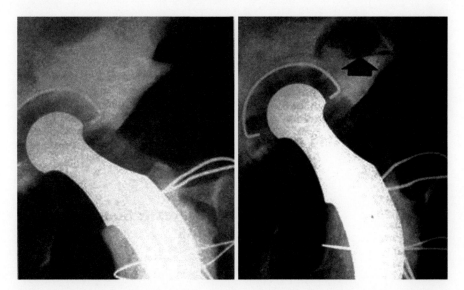

Figs. 11.3 and 11.4 Radiograph showing cavitation around the cement peg in the acetabulum

On the femoral side a loose stem or stem-cement complex, may act as a piston. When combined with a mechanical situation of a one-way non-return valve effect, it is easy to appreciate that an increase in intramedullary pressure may become symptomatic under load. This mechanism of cyclic pressure changes could explain endosteal cavitation.

In summary: If we accept that freedom from pain after total hip arthroplasty is because the natural symptomatic, is replaced with artificial neuropathic, we must accept the corollary: failure of the artificial can only present clinically through its effect on the natural.

References

1. Wroblewski BM. Pain in osteoarthritis of the hip. Practitioner. 1978;Jan:140–1.
2. Hodgkinson JP, Shelley P, Wroblewski BM. The correlation between the roentgenographic appearance and the operative findings at the bone-cement junction of the socket in Charnley low friction arthroplasties. Clin Orthop. 1988;228:105–9.
3. Wroblewski BM, Fleming PA, Siney PD. Charnley low-friction torque arthroplasty of the hip. 20–30 year results. J Bone Joint Surg (Br). 1999;81-B:427–30.
4. Harris WH, McCarthy JC, O'Neill DA. Femoral component loosening using contemporary techniques of femoral cement fixation. J Bone Joint Surg (Am). 1982;64-A:1063–7.
5. Wroblewski BM, Siney PD, Fleming PA. Wear and fracture of acetabular cup in Charnley low-friction arthroplasty. J Arthroplasty. 1998;13(2):132–7.

Chapter 12
Pulmonary Embolism After Total Hip Arthroplasty

Total hip replacement offers a very important field for studying this complication (pulmonary embolism) *because it is performed in relatively large numbers on a small range of closely related hip conditions.*

Embolism following total hip replacement presents a special problem because to achieve full anticoagulant levels quickly brings risks of wound haematoma… and invites infection

Fatal pulmonary embolism is rightly considered the most serious event, more so when it occurs after elective surgery for a condition that, by itself, is not life threatening. The advent of total hip arthroplasty, as a method of choice of treatment for the arthritic hip, has uncovered the demand, extended the indications and increased the expectations of an ever more favourable outcome. The emphasis has changed from pain relief to activity levels demanded or promised.

It is, therefore, not unexpected that under such circumstances single adverse events attract wide publicity and focus the attention on the all encompassing term: thromboprophylaxis.

The literature on the ever changing subject of thromboprophylaxis is so vast that any attempt to offer even a summary would not do justice.

Increasingly more sophisticated methods of the diagnosis, prevention and treatment, demand ever greater numbers in any study to establish a level of statistically acceptable significance.

Whether the results in such studies make an individual clinician's decision any easier is debatable: "We think in generalities but we live in detail" (Alfred North Whitehead 1861–1947).

It is probably correct to suggest that the general perception is that prevention of clot formation is not only possible but mandatory. The pressure on clinicians is to apply the currently applicable "thromboprophylactic measures" for to do otherwise might imply negligence. Under such circumstances complications of the "prophylaxis" are, at times, more readily acceptable.

© Springer International Publishing Switzerland 2016
B.M. Wroblewski et al., *Charnley Low-Frictional Torque Arthroplasty of the Hip:
Practice and Results*, DOI 10.1007/978-3-319-21320-0_12

In clinical practice three aspects remain of importance:

- Circumstances leading to clot formation.
- Events resulting in clot migration.
- The consequences.

Clot Formation

In this context the Virchows's triad is usually quoted [1]. The three factors predisposing to intravascular thrombosis are:

- Alterations of patterns of blood flow
- Damage to the vascular endothelium.
- Changes in blood constituents – hypercoagulability.

Prevention of clot formation would obviate the need for any more complex measures to be applied. The assumption is not only simple but may appear very logical: Unfortunately – by definition – what does not clot – bleeds.

Clot Migration

The clot, once formed, must be the subject of Newton's First law of motion "it must be ácted upon by an external force" in order to move from its position of rest.

The clot at risk for migration would be the one that is not firmly adherent to the vessel wall. Therefore more likely formed in larger veins, with larger calibre vessels downstream from the clot. Compressive stockings may encourage venous return or help to prevent clot migration, once the clot has formed. Early mobilisation may help to prevent clot formation, but may encourage clot migration once the clot has formed.

The Consequences

The consequences of clot migration? A spectrum from the asymptomatic to fatal. This is related to the mass of the clot. This is the most urgent and clinically significant event.

The long-term effects on the pulmonary circulation have not received detailed attention. This is either because the mild episodes do not carry significant long-term problems, or conversely they make take years to present clinically. Even if, or when they do, such patients are unlikely to find themselves under the care of an orthopaedic surgeon. Pulmonary hypertension has not been a subject of investigations. From long-term follow-up studies, it would appear that some 18–22 years must elapse before a previously well documented deep vein thrombosis presented as a local venous insufficiency [2].

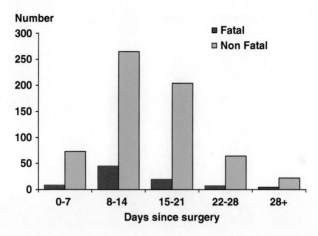

Fig. 12.1 Fatal and non fatal pulmonary embolism. Time of occurrence of pulmonary embolism in relation to the operation of hip replacement

Studies of Post-operative Pulmonary Embolism

Results of the studies of post-operative pulmonary embolism are better understood when the clinical experience and practice are taken into account. There was caution concerning early mobilization and no pressure for early discharge. Reliance was on clinical acumen, autopsies were almost routine and carried out in the Hospital. It could be argued that the post-operative routine would carry higher incidence of the complications. This may be so, but does early discharge merely moves the responsibility for the correct diagnosis from the Hospital to District? What chance that a death after discharge be reported as due to myocardial infarction?

Johnson and Charnley (1977) [3] studied prophylaxis, incidence and treatment of pulmonary embolism during the 12 year period, 1962–1973, when 7959 LFAs have been carried out.

Clinical evidence of non-fatal pulmonary embolism was found in 628 (7.9 %) of patients. In that group 127 (20.2 %) had clinical evidence of deep vein thrombosis. By contrast in the group of 83 patients (1.04 %) who had fatal pulmonary embolism, only one had clinical evidence of deep vein thrombosis. The suggestion is that the thrombi that are most likely to embolise are either formed centrally, or if formed distally, they do not cause sufficient venous obstruction so as to present clinically.

Johnson et al. (1977) [4] used the above-quoted study [3] to establish the incidence of pulmonary embolism with respect to the operation.

The results are shown in Fig. 12.1 Over 70 % of both the fatal and the non-fatal emboli occurred in the second and third week after the operation.

The findings have very significant practical implications. Early mobilisation and discharge may help prevent clot formation but may not give a true incidence of clot migration – embolism. Careful monitoring after discharge is essential.

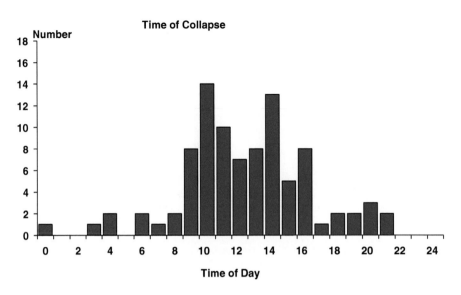

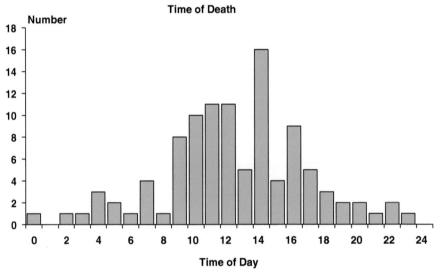

Fig. 12.2 Fatal pulmonary embolism – diurnal variations. Time of day when collapse and death occurred

Fatal Pulmonary Embolism: Diurnal Variations

During the 17 year period 1970–1986, 18,104 Charnley LFAs had been carried out at Wrightington Hospital. There were 122 deaths (0.67 %) from pulmonary embolism; 71 % confirmed by post-mortem examination. The time at risk was 9.00 am to 4.00 pm and accounted for 82 % of cases; 86 % of patients were mobilising and 70.2 % died within 1 h of collapse [5] (Fig. 12.2).

Fatal Pulmonary Embolism After Revision of Failed Total Hip Arthroplasty

In this group of patients, mobilisation was delayed for up to 3 weeks. In 1483 consecutive revisions there were 54 cases (3.6 %) of pulmonary embolism diagnosed clinically. There were six deaths (0.4 %) all submitted to post-mortem examination. There was one death from pulmonary embolism (0.07 %). This occurred on the day of revision in an 88 year old male who was referred following periprosthetic fracture of the femur sustained 3 weeks previously. He had suffered a recent stroke and was known to have bronchial carcinoma [6].

Seasonal Variation of Fatal Pulmonary Embolism

The material for the study of diurnal variations was also used to examine suspected seasonal variations in the incidence of fatal pulmonary embolism. There was statistically significant variation in the seasonal incidence of fatal pulmonary embolism. This was 1 % from November through to February compared with 0.42 % for the remainder of the year [7] (Fig. 12.3).

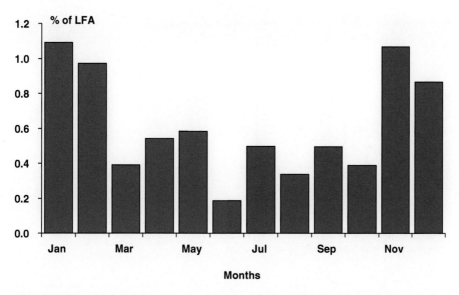

Fig. 12.3 Seasonal variation of fatal pulmonary embolism. Winter months have a higher incidence

Seasonal Variations. The Effect of Atmospheric Conditions

With the availability of very detailed data the opportunity was taken to examine a possible effect of atmospheric conditions – humidity and pressure – on the incidence of fatal pulmonary embolism. Three-hourly recordings of atmospheric pressure and humidity over the 17-year period were examined with correction for the elevation of the Hospital above sea level. No statistical evidence of correlation was found. However, the **rate of change** of both atmospheric pressure and humidity was significantly higher during the episodes when fatal pulmonary emboli were recorded.

If mechanical reasons for clot migration are accepted, then it could be argued that the rapid change in atmospheric pressure acts as either a pressure or decompression mechanism altering the venous capacity and the rate of flow and hence clot migration (Fig. 12.4).

Changes in humidity could have the same effect through rate of peripheral blood flow in controlling body temperature by diverting the venous blood flow from the central or the peripheral circulation (Fig. 12.5).

Prevention of clot formation may be within clinical control – clot migration, embolism, may not.

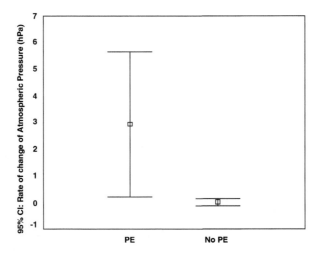

Fig. 12.4 Atmospheric Pressure. Comparison of the rate of change when fatal pulmonary embolism occurred with times free from such fatalities

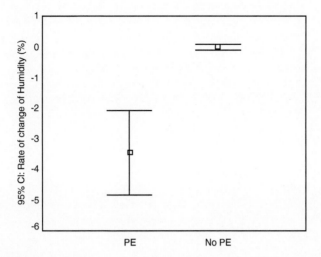

Fig. 12.5 Humidity. Comparison of the rate of change when fatal pulmonary embolism occurred with times free from such fatalities

References

1. Carter AE, Elban R. Prevention of postoperative deep vein thrombosis in legs by administered hydroxychloroquine sulphate. Br Med J. 1974;3:94.
2. Chrisman OD, Snook GA, Wilson TC, Short JY. Prevention of venous thromboembolism by administration of hydroxychloroquine. J Bone Joint Surg. (Am) 1976;58A:918.
3. Johnson R, Charnley J. Treatment of pulmonary embolism in total hip replacement. Clin Orthop. 1977;124:149–54.
4. Johnson R, Green JR, Charnley J. Pulmonary embolism and its prophylaxis following the Charnley total hip replacement. Clin Orthop. 1977;127:123–32.
5. Wroblewski BM, Siney PD, Fleming PA. Fatal pulmonary embolism after total hip arthroplasty: diurnal variations. Orthopaedics. 1998;12:1269–71.
6. Wroblewski BM, Siney PD, Fleming PA, Kay P. Fatal pulmonary embolism and mortality after revision of failed total hip arthroplasties. J Arthroplast. 2000;15:437–9.
7. Wroblewski BM, Siney PD, Fleming PA, Kay P. Seasonal variations in the incidence of fatal pulmonary embolism. The effect of atmospheric conditions. Clin Orthop. 1992;276:222–4.

Part II
Deep Infection

Chapter 13
Deep Infection

Deep Infection [1]

We define deep infection as – infection around the implant.

The most likely source of infection that was not under control by standard aseptic precautions appeared to be the air of the operating room. It was therefore decided to build a clean air operating enclosure.

"The general opinion would seem to be that the air of an average operating theatre is relatively innocuous. In the ward, on the other hand, the aerial route for post-operative cross-infection is regarded as potent…" "This was the opinion I myself held until some two years ago when a very high rate of wound infection in a new type of arthroplasty prompted this study" (1964).

Post-operative sepsis, resulting in the infection around the implant, during the years 1958–1967, was so high (8.9 %) that it would have been necessary to abandon this type of surgery had not special precautions in the operating theatre shown a marked improvement.

A prototype filtered air enclosure was constructed to contain the lower half of the patient's body and the three surgeons of the operating team. Filtered air is forced in at the top of the enclosure and the surgeons wear respirators through which their exhaled air is extracted so as not to mix with the filtered air of the enclosure. (1964) (Fig 13.1).

The First Survey

The study related to 2170 consecutive arthroplasties of the hip joint performed between January 1959 and September 1967 (Table 13.1, Fig. 13.2) "… *to permit at least 12 months to elapse between the last operation and completing the report.*"

© Springer International Publishing Switzerland 2016
B.M. Wroblewski et al., *Charnley Low-Frictional Torque Arthroplasty of the Hip: Practice and Results*, DOI 10.1007/978-3-319-21320-0_13

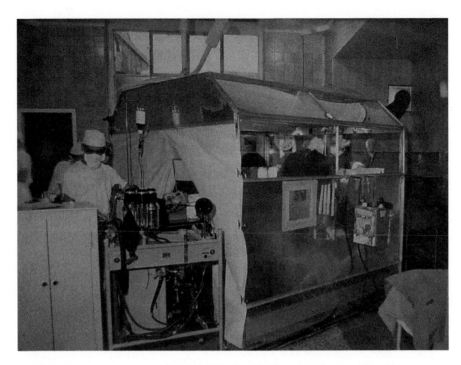

Fig. 13.1 The original clean air enclosure "the Greenhouse" at Wrightington Hospital

Table 13.1 Study of infection after low-frictional torque arthoplasties – Jan 1959 to Sept 1967 and subsequently (Fig. 13.2)

Phase	Period	Operating room	Colonies per plate per hour	No. of hip replacements	Infection rate %
1	Jan 1959 to Nov 1961	Primitive	80–90	190	8.9
2	Nov 1961 to June 1962	Prototype filtered air enclosure 10 air changes per hour	2.5	108	3.7
3	June 1962 to March 1966	Clean air enclosure 130 air changes per hour	1.9	1164	2.2
4	June 1966 to Sept. 1967	Clean air enclosure 300 air changes per hour	Air not sterile Lowest that can be recorded	708	1.3
5	1969 -	As above Total body exhaust suits	Lowest recorded	1000	1.0

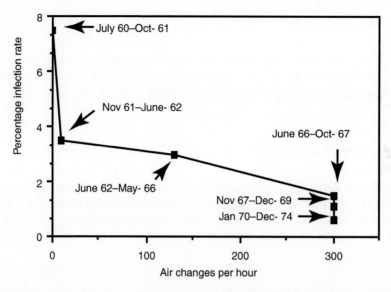

Fig. 13.2 Graph of infection rates. The study related to 2170 consecutive arthroplasties of the hip joint performed between January 1959 and September 1967. Further information was added to 1974 (Reproduced from Wroblewski [10])

"*It was not possible to exclude a number of additional variables which could contribute to a reduction in wound infection … improved form of wound closure … the bodies of the surgeons or the others in the operating team, through permeability of the textile gowns.*" "*Though the filtered air enclosure has improved the air cleanliness 25 times … it is still not completely sterile. It would be unlikely that a total abolition of infection could be expected.*" "*Despite extreme precautions our rate is still about 1.8 %*" (1968).

It was in the early stages of the development of the clean air operating enclosure (1964) "*… another line … A form of 'air curtain' in which the enclosure acts as a hood or shield to reduce the tendency of the cold air flow to entrain infected particles.*" Charnley was clearly considering the next stage in the development of clean air enclosure – without side panels, pointing out that this "*… will effect an economy in the volume of air required and necessitate in the method of illumination.*"

The complexity of the problem becomes obvious when one considers numbers of operations, diagnostic criteria, follow-up, and the time interval from the primary operation to establishing the diagnosis of deep infection.

Establishing the Diagnosis

Clinical experience suggests that establishing the diagnosis of deep infection is easier in cases referred for a second opinion than after our own operations.

Clinical Diagnosis

Pain relief after THA is such a consistent feature that failure to relieve pain must put the surgeon on guard. Barring any problems at surgery there are only three possibilities: inappropriate indication, inappropriate patient selection, infection.

Inappropriate Indication

Clinical assessment fails to identify the source of pain. The radiograph is viewed before, or at the same time, as taking the history and examining the patient. Clinical assessment must come before viewing radiographs; radiographs merely confirm and offer a record of what is usually obvious from the history and examination.

Inappropriate Patient Selection

It must not be assumed that every patient with an arthritic hip would benefit from THA. Rare though it may, beware of a patient with a very high expectation and flattering the surgeon's apparent skill and reputation. Does the surgeon's ability match patient's expectations? It must not be assumed that to do something is to do good, while to advise delaying surgery implies unwillingness to help, or negligence.

Complications

Dislocation is obvious, loosening of components comes later and is largely asymptomatic, fracture of the stem is now a late rarity – that leaves infection.

History of haematoma, delayed wound healing, courses of antibiotics – increase the index of suspicion. Regular follow-up with good quality radiographs and continuity of observer method is essential.

Bacteriology in the study of deep infection after THA is outside the scope of this work. It is best left in the hands of the experts on the subject.

Classification of Deep Infection

The practical usefulness of any classification is inversely proportional to its complexity. Infection will continue to be studied retrospectively if meaningful information is to be gathered.

Early Infection

Signs of inflammation, delayed would healing, infected haematoma, purulent discharge and early sinus formation. Wound dehiscence of deep fascia is extremely rare. Early exploration under conditions as in the primary operation, evacuation, examination of the deep fascia for deep extension, but without probing or opening unless communication is obvious.

Charnley arranged for photographs of the wounds to be taken before discharge from the hospital: 5400 photographs are available for further studies to anyone interested in the subject.

Late diagnosis of early infection is probably the most common scenario. Delays or lack of follow-up, inadequate radiographs, and lack of awareness of the possibility of infection.

Late presentation following early contamination. This is a complex subject that continues to be debated. If this is a true entity in clinical practice then fortunately it has not presented itself, as would have been expected, with increasing follow-up.

Late haematogenous infection – fortunately very rare. The criteria for the diagnosis must be strict: Primary surgery in a patient not at risk, no post-operative complications suggesting a possibility of infection. Clinical success with normal radiographs – well documented over a period of probably not <3 years, a source of possible bacteraemia, for example lower limb skin infection.

Establishing the Incidence

Deep infection after THA is rightly considered a very serious complication. Other than being a disappointment both to the patient and the surgeon, it brings with it the added socio-economic problems. It is, therefore, not surprising that so much effort has been put in by Charnley not only to identify and, if possible, eliminate the sources of infection, but also develop methods to reduce the chances of wound contamination. With deep infection rate reduced to about 1 %, efforts to establish infection rate – in general – has become a complex issue; increasing effort – diminishing return.

The Size of Sample Under Review

It is suggested that the value of any study of deep infection after THA is proportional to the size of the sample and the length of follow-up. This sets the limit on a particular unit to be able to provide "numbers" and suggests multi-centre studies. Multi-centre studies bring with them the problems of variations in patient selection, theatre environment, surgical technique, prophylactic measures, criteria of establishing the diagnosis, but above all, good quality records – and of course availability of follow-up.

Since no single case is likely to be recorded more than once, conversely loss of one case, where the incidence is very low, will have a significant effect.

The Length of Follow-Up

Deep infection after this operation can never be overlooked … if sufficient time is allowed to elapse. (1969)

Infection with dehiscence of the wound and skin – implant communication is extremely rare. More common, but still rare, is the sequence of: delayed wound healing followed by apparent success – both clinical and radiological – at least for a period of time. Detailed history and good quality radiographs are invaluable.

In case where deep infection is eventually confirmed, they offer very useful material for retrospective reviews and learning material for future interpretations.

As an example, Van Niekerk and Charnley (1979) studied the incidence of infection in a group of 2154 cases operated upon during a 2 year period: Jan 1974–Jan 1976. Deep infection was reported as 0.3 % – a remarkably low incidence. Caution is essential in interpreting the results. Not only was the follow-up relatively short but **infection was confirmed by bacteriology at revision** [2]. The information indicates that any infected arthroplasty that has not been revised, or where cultures failed to produce a growth of an organism, were excluded. This would possibly explain the very low incidence. In a further study the results of 1542 LFAs, carried out over an 8 year period, were reviewed with a minimum follow-up of 2 years. Deep infection was recorded as 1.5 % [3].

Since a number of cases of spontaneous healing of deep infection have not attracted attention it is probably correct to suggest that: given time, infection will declare itself. Although 1 year may be sufficient, with good quality records and frequent follow-up, ideally a 2–4 years period is probably more realistic.

Patients at Risk for Deep Infection [4]

The analysis relates to cases which were technically much more difficult as well as more prone to infection.

Failures of Previous Hip Operations

Between November 1962 and April 1969, 203 patients had undergone 217 LFAs for failures of previous hip operations (Table 13.2). They reflect a spectrum of operative procedures that had been in common use until the advent of the LFA. Plain acrylic cement was used in all cases.

Table 13.2 Previous hip operations in 203 patients, 217 LFAs

Previous operation	Number
Femoral osteotomy	121
Hemiarthroplasty	51
Other: Cup arthroplasty	17
Pseudarthrosis	9
Arthrodesis	9
Total hip replacement (Not LFA)	10
Total	217

A review of the results of 217 LFAs carried out in 1971/1972 emphasised some aspects of the technique, the clinical results as well as infection rate. Eight patients (3.7 %) developed wound infection: four early and four after the first year [4].

Urethral Instrumentation After LFA

One hundred and ninety five males had urinary retention in the immediate post-operative period requiring insertion of urethral catheter and, at times, prostatectomy. Twelve, 6.2 % developed deep infection around the hip implant [5]. "Catheter fever" is a well documented complication of urethral instrumentation.

(It may be of interest to put it on record that when the operation, the LFA, was first introduced as a routine procedure, all patients had catheter insertion pre-operatively. The objective was to avoid possible perforation of the bladder during the preparation of the acetabulum using the perforating, deepening and expanding acetabular reamers).

Diabetic Patient

There was a low representation of diabetic patients because selection was prejudiced against diabetics for this type of surgery.

A retrospective review of 62 LFAs in 44 diabetic patients has shown a superficial wound infection rate of 9.7 %; deep infection rate was 5.6 % – with a follow-up of 1–7.5 years.

The conclusion was: antibiotic prophylaxis should be part of the routine practice [6].

Patients with Psoriasis

Retrospective review of 55 LFAs in 38 patients with established psoriasis has shown a superficial infection rate of 9.1 % and a deep infection rate of 5.5 % with a follow-up of 1–12 years. Antibiotic prophylaxis is indicated in patients with psoriasis undergoing LFA [7].

A summary of patients at risk for deep infection can be seen in Table 13.3.

Table 13.3 Summary of results in patients at risk for deep infection

Patients at risk	Number of LFAs	Follow-up years	% Infection
Previous hip surgery	217	5	7.6
Urethral instrumentation	195	2.1	6.2
Diabetes	62	1–7.5	5.6
Psoriasis	55	1–12	5.5

Table 13.4 Time to revision after primary LFA

Time to revision (years)	Number of LFAs	% of Revisions
1–4	147	59
5–10	71	28.5
10+	31	12.5
Total	249	100 %

Late Haematogenous Infection

Deep infection after this operation can never be overlooked … if sufficient time is allowed to elapse.

Late haematogenous infection is not a topic of frequent reports other than single sporadic cases. The reason for this probably stems from the very definition and the criteria that must be fulfilled to identify such cases. Included must only be the patients undergoing primary operations, not at a risk for infection, having had well documented successful clinical and radiographic evidence of success, and a continuous follow-up for a number of years yet to be specified. Late diagnosis of early infection must be excluded and late clinical presentation of contamination, during the primary operation, must also be considered.

Results

To offer some indication of the complexity of this topic the details are given below:

During the 43 year period 1962–2005, 22,066 Charnley LFAs had been carried out at Wrightington Hospital. During that time 249–1.13 % had been revised for deep infection. The timing of the revisions are shown in Table 13.4.

Of the 31 revisions for deep infection carried out after 10 years or more, 11 are analysed in some detail in Table 13.5. (This is merely an attempt to highlight the complexity of the issue; the availability of good quality records is immediately obvious).

Rare though this may be, late haematogenous infection must always be considered as a possible cause of long-term failure.

With increasing numbers of young patients accepted for this type of surgery, increasing possibility of long-term problems is to be expected. Continuity of well structured follow-up facilities must be part of the original consent for the operation.

Table 13.5 Details of 11 cases revised for late haematogenous infection

Follow-up (years)	Source of infection suspected/ identified	Bacteriology at revision	Comment
31	Infected total knee (ipsilateral)	Staph epidermidis	Antibiotics Before revision
22	Abcess behind knee (ipsilateral)	Staph aureus	Fractured stem
18	Infected bunion (contralateral)	Haemolytic strep Staph aureus	Antibiotic Before revision
15	Bladder surgery for neoplasia	Staph epidermidis	Antibiotic Before revision
11	Dental abcess	Negative	Antibiotic Before revision
10	Bacterial endocarditis	Streptococcus	Antibiotic Before revision
10	Compound fracture dislocation of finger	Staph aureus	Diabetic
18 Bilateral	Bilateral infections Dislocation left Source unknown	Staph aureus	Trochanteric Non-union
12	Source unknown	Coag. neg. staph	
11	Source unknown	Coag. neg. staph Acinetobacter	Heavy fall

Deep Infection: Theatre Gowns

> *Bacteriological tests show that the fine woven material … used extensively for operating gowns, can be penetrated by the organisms from surgeon's body*

Charnley Total Body Exhaust Suits (Fig. 13.3)

Although the introduction of clean air enclosure, total body exhaust suits and the instrument tray system have reduced the infection rate from 8.9 % to about 1 %, infection was not eliminated altogether. It was essential to identify further possible sources of wound contamination which may lead to infection. Charnley and Eftekhar [8] studied permeability of the surgical gowns which were in common use. Their suspicions were confirmed: bacteria did penetrate the surgeon's gowns. One further source of possible wound contamination was established. Attention could now be directed towards alternative, non-permeable materials for the gowns. The findings also *"offered an explanation that operations which were unusually difficult technically and require unusually physical effort, tend more often to be followed by infection than do simple operations."* Physical exertion generating movement and heat, glove-gown-wound contact, plus tissue damage and prolonged exposure of the operation site all contribute to the possibility of infection.

Fig. 13.3 The original
Charnley total body
exhaust suits

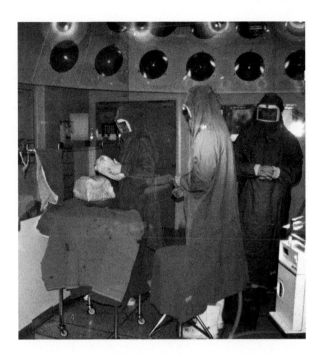

Charnley and Eftekhar also stated: *"The more impermeable the material of the surgeon's gown the more the surgeon needs to have a cooling system to take away the very considerable amount of heat generated in strenuous orthopaedic operations."*

For the detailed description of the design and function of the Body Exhaust System the reader must reference Charnley's book: Low Friction Arthroplasty of the Hip – Theory and Practice [9].

Disposable Gowns and Ventilated Helmets

The recent introduction of disposable gowns and ventilated helmets poses a number of questions:

–   Is the independently powered fan which is a part of the helmet, powerful enough to counteract up-currents to expel the air to the ground level; not only at rest but also during the physical exertion at surgery?
–   Is the air introduced into the helmet merely mixed with the up-currents and the exhaled air, and forced out through the nearest "escape routes"?
–   Is the benefit primarily for the surgeon's comfort than the safety of the patient?

Here we have a very fertile ground for research.

Comment

It is essential to understand the principle underlying the design and function of the total body exhaust suits. The Charnley system is designed to protect the operation site and the clean air enclosure from contamination by the operating team.

The suction system extracts the air from within the gowns and disposes it outside the operating theatre. The air flow follows the pressure gradient: from the clean air, into the exhaust suits and to the outside.

The self-contained pressure suit system takes the clean air from the operating theatre, filters it further by the helmet filter, and delivers it to the inside of the suit.

The airflow will follow the pressure gradient from within the gowns into the clean air enclosure through the nearest available exits. Whether the system is powerful enough to overcome the up-currents generated by the bodies of the operating team and deposit it at the floor level is debatable.

Is the system designed to offer personal protection for the wearer? Any risk to the operating team from the clean air theatre environment is yet to be documented. A higher infection rate should not come as a surprise.

References

1. Charnley J. Post operative infection after total hip replacement with special reference to air contamination in the operating room. Clin Orthop Relat Res. 1972;87:167–87.
2. Van Niekerk GA, Charnley J. Post-operative infection after Charnley low-friction arthroplasty of the hip. Internal publication No: 68. Centre for Hip Surgery, Wrightington Hospital; 1977.
3. Lynch M, Esser MP, Shelley P, Wroblewski BM. Deep infection in Charnley low friction arthroplasty. J Bone Joint Surg. 1987;69-B:355–60.
4. Dupont JA, Charnley J. Low friction arthroplasty of the hip for failures of previous operations. J Bone Joint Surg (Br). 1972;54B:77–87.
5. Wroblewski BM, Del Sel HJ. Urethral instrumentation and deep sepsis in total hip replacement. Clin Orthop Rel Res. 1980;146:209–1.
6. Menon TJ, Thjellesen D, Wroblewski BM. Charnley low-friction arthroplasty in diabetic patients. J Bone Joint Surg (Br). 1983;65-B:580–1.
7. Menon TJ, Wroblewski BM. Charnley low-friction arthroplasty in patients with psoriasis. Clin Orthop Rel Res. 1983;176:127–8.
8. Charnley J, Eftekhar N. Postoperative infection in total prosthetic replacement arthroplasty of the hip joint with special reference to the bacterial content of the air of the operating room. J Bone Joint Surg (Br). 1969;56-B:45–9.
9. Charnley J. Low friction arthroplasty of the hip. Theory and practice. Berlin: Springer Verlag; 1979. p. 173–9.
10. Wroblewski BM. Revision surgery in total hip arthroplasty. London: Springer Verlag; 1990.

Chapter 14
Deep Infection: The Role of Acrylic Cement

When the infection rate was high, in the early years of this study, this cement was used only for the femoral prosthesis, but after 1961 the amount of cement doubled, being used for the socket as well, and despite this infection rates continued to fall.

Plain acrylic cement (CMW Laboratories now DePuy International, Blackpool, U.K.) was used in all cases. At one stage cement was suspected to be a contributory factor responsible for high infection rates. Because antibiotics were not included in the cement it was possible to establish the benefit of clean air enclosure, total body exhaust system and the instrument trays in reducing the infection rates. Use of cement was not the factor contributing to deep infection.

Antibiotic Containing Acrylic Cement

Buchholz and Colleagues [1] were the first to introduce antibiotic containing acrylic cement. Palacos/Gentamicin combination, was used both for prevention of deep infection in primary surgery and in one-stage revisions for deep infection. The release of Gentamicin was measured by its concentration in blood, urine, adjacent tissues and wound drainage fluid.

From various studies the conclusion was that Gentamicin does leach out from acrylic cement and that it is useful in reducing infection rate in primary procedures and also offering a high success rate in one-stage revisions for deep infection.

© Springer International Publishing Switzerland 2016
B.M. Wroblewski et al., *Charnley Low-Frictional Torque Arthroplasty of the Hip: Practice and Results*, DOI 10.1007/978-3-319-21320-0_14

Table 14.1 Comparison of results, with respect to deep infection, with plain CMW, and Gentamicin containing Palacos acrylic cement

	CMW Plain			Palacos + Gentamicin		
	Number	Follow up (years)	Infection %	Number	Follow up (years)	Infection %
O.A.	599	7.6	1.5	395	3.2	1.5
Rh. A.	41	7.6	4.9	29	2.6	3.5
Previous surgery	125	9.2	4.0	55	3.5	1.8
THA & hemi	106	7.8	2.8	192	3.1	0.5
All cases with previous operation	231	8.5	3.5	247	3.2	0.8
Primary LFA	640	7.6	1.7	424	2.9	1.7

Comparison of Results Using Plain and Gentamicin Acrylic Cement [2]

Once the value of clean air enclosure, total body exhaust suits and the instrument tray system had been established, the next step was to examine the contribution that Gentamicin containing acrylic cement would make.

A retrospective review of 1542 Charnley LFAs was carried out. This was a single surgeon series. The operations were carried out during an 8 year period 1976–1983 and reviewed in 1987 to allow reasonable follow-up (Table 14.1).

Conclusions

- The overall infection rate was 2.18 % in the plain acrylic cement group and 1.34 % in the Gentamicin containing group – the difference is not statistically significant.
- In the primary operations the deep infection rate was comparable 1.72 % and 1.7 %.
- In secondary operations Gentamicin containing acrylic cement gave significantly better results: 0.8 % infection rate compared with 3.5 %.
- Radiological diagnosis of deep infection, after the primary operation, was possible within 1 year of surgery in all cases except one. In this single case deep infection followed an infected skin lesion on the ipsilateral leg which occurred in the fourth post-operative year and must be regarded as late haematogenous infection.
- Addition of Gentamicin to acrylic cement had no significant effect on reducing deep infection rate in primary procedures over and above that achieved with clean air enclosure, total body exhaust suits and the instrument tray system, but was of benefit in secondary operations.

Release of Gentamicin from Acrylic Cement: An Ex-Vivo Study [3]

A different approach, to estimate the amount of antibiotic released from cement, was called for. If the amount of antibiotic included in the cement is known and the concentration assumed to be uniform, then examining the cement removed at revision surgery would give some indication of the antibiotic retained and thus the amount of antibiotic released. Sixteen cases were included in the study. All were revisions of failed THA where Palacos acrylic cement with Gentamicin had been used in the primary operation. At revision extracted cement was assayed for Gentamicin levels. The technical details of the assays can be found in the original publication [3].

The conclusions were:

- On average 78 % (55–98 %) of Gentamicin was retained within the acrylic cement.
- The amount of Gentamicin released was, on average, 2 mgm (milligrams) (1–3.4 mgm) per gram of polymerised cement.
- Assuming that the whole 80 g of cement was used for the operation (40 g for the cup and 40 g for the stem) then the total amount of Gentamicin released about 160 mgm (8–272 mgm) would have been available. Assuming a 40 mgm as a single dose then (0.5–7) doses would have been delivered locally.
- There was no great variation in the amount of Gentamicin released during the 1–48 month period.

Summary of Conclusions

- Release from acrylic cement occurs early – probably within days.
- The amount released is proportional to the surface area of the cement.
- The release is neither continuous nor complete on average: 78 % of Gentamicin remains within the cement.
- The combination of cement/antibiotic mixtures could be expected to offer additional protection to clean air enclosure, total body exhaust suits, instrument tray system, patient selection and adequate surgical technique.
- Indication for the use: patients known to be at risk for infection and revisions.

Leaching Out from Acrylic Cement [4]

Theoretical Consideration and Practical Evaluation

Inclusion of an antibiotic in acrylic cement must take into account the characteristics of the antibiotic and the nature of the cement. The antibiotics must be heat stable as not to be inactivated by the heat of cement polymerisation, as well as be soluble in tissue fluids to allow the release of the antibiotic from the cement. Common salt (NaCl) fulfils the criteria.

Extensive experiments, in vitro, using common salt and CMW plain cement have shown that for any concentration the amount of common salt released from the cement was proportional to the surface area of the cement. Clearly, in clinical practice the area of the bone-cement contact must be far greater than can be reproduced in laboratory experiments; the basic conclusion, however, is correct. The model offers the opportunity to study "patterns of release" from polymerised cement.

Release from Polymerized Acrylic Cement: A Practical Demonstration

The physical characteristics of antibiotic release from polymerised cement can be demonstrated using Gentian Violet (hexamethylpararosanilinechloride) and a solution of a bleach containing 3–6 % sodium hypochlorite (Figs. 14.1 and 14.2).

Conclusion

A smooth, glass-like finish allows release of only the material at the very surface of the cement. Inclusions at the subsurface are not released. By contrast, an irregular rough cement mass offers a larger surface area, a more extensive ingress of the bleaching agent (or tissue fluids in clinical practice) and, therefore, greater release of Gentian Violet (or antibiotic in clinical practice).

These findings have clinical implications. If the objective of cement spacers is to offer antibiotic release in the first stage revision then injection moulded, smooth surface including articulating spacers, are most unsuitable.

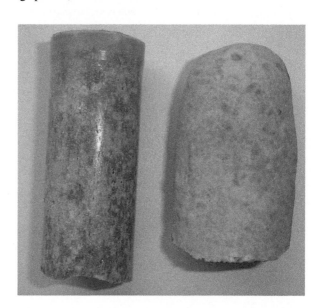

Fig. 14.1 Cement after bleaching. On the *left*: Injection moulded cement with a smooth surface finish showing patchy areas of bleaching. On the *right*: cement with an irregular rough finish with more extensive bleaching

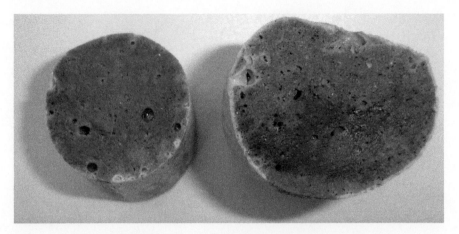

Fig. 14.2 Cement after bleaching. On the *left*: Injection moulded cement. On the *right*: cement with an irregular rough finish. Deeper layers are not bleached in both specimens. This demonstrates the limitations of cement spacers for antibiotic release

The cost implications of each method must also be taken into consideration.

Antibiotic Containing Cement Spacers [5]

A two-stage revision of infected total joint replacement appears to be the accepted method. The first stage includes, among others, the insertion of antibiotic containing cement spacer. The detailed analysis of the method is outside this brief comment.

Our limited experience with this method dates back to 1982 [5] when antibiotic containing cement spacer was used to fill up the gap and stabilise the pseudarthrosis after removal of an infected total knee replacement. In four cases the method was successful at a mean follow-up of 36.4 months, the longest remains symptom free at 24 years. The method was used out of clinical necessity for individual patients, at the time of the operation.

References

1. Buchholz HW, Engelbrecht H. Uber die Depotwirkung einiger Antibiotica bei Vermischung mit dem Kunstharz Palacos. Chirurg. 1970;41:511–5.
2. Lynch M, Esser MP, Shelley P, Wroblewski BM. Comparison of plain and gentamicin loaded acrylic cement. J Bone Joint Surg (Br). 1987;69-B:355–60.
3. Wroblewski BM, Esser M, Srigley DW. Release of Gentamicin from acrylic bone cement. An ex-vivo study. Acta Orthop Scand. 1986;57:413–4.
4. Wroblewski BM. Leaching out from acrylic bone-cement. Experimental evaluation. Clin Orthop Rel Res. 1979;124:311.
5. Jones WA, Wroblewski BM. Salvage of failed total knee arthroplasty: the "beefburger" procedure. J Bone Joint Surg (Br). 1998;71-B:856–7.

Chapter 15
Management of Deep Infection

Deep infection after elective surgery is a serious complication. The problem is even more serious when a large foreign body, an implant, is an integral part of the original treatment.

In the management of deep infection after total hip arthroplasty the work of Buchholz and Colleagues has made an original and very valuable contribution: the use of antibiotic containing acrylic cement (ACAC). With time, increasing numbers of publications on the subject appeared in print. The method advocated by Buchholz and Colleagues, one stage revision, did not become readily accepted despite encouraging results. The reason is by no means clear. Was it the fear of exacerbation of the infection, the length of the operative procedure, or merely the lack of stamina on the part of the surgeon and the operating team?

One Stage Revision: The Principle [1–3]

Operative intervention in cases of infection, in any site, follows well documented principles: Removal of foreign material, if present, clearing of all infected tissues and exposing healthy deeper tissues – (as much as technically possible), application of local antiseptics/antibiotics, closure of cavities, ensuring mechanical stability, drainage of the site, rest for the patient as well as of the part involved, antibiotics. Thus the question whether the new implant is inserted has not been considered, it has been expressly implied as part of the accepted principles:

Local Antibiotics: ACAC filling the cavities thus ensuring largest possible surface area of antibiotic elution.

Closure of cavities – of the medullary canal and the acetabulum: Total hip arthroplasty components with ACAC offer not only the closure of the cavities but also stability to the site.

© Springer International Publishing Switzerland 2016   127
B.M. Wroblewski et al., *Charnley Low-Frictional Torque Arthroplasty of the Hip: Practice and Results*, DOI 10.1007/978-3-319-21320-0_15

To reach that stage clearance of both the foreign and infected materials becomes the most demanding part of the procedure – demanding of time and detailed performance.

The implantation of the new components becomes just another "primary" procedure – one of several on the particular operation day. In a study of 183 THAs revised for deep infection in a one-stage procedure, over 85 % of patients were free of infection at an average follow-up of 7.9 years [4].

Two Stage Revision

The principle of two stage revision follows the same operative routine up to but not including the implantation of the new components. It is at that stage that ACAC "spacers" are used to deliver local antibiotics. The spacers do not fill the cavities as intimately as fully pressurised cement can, neither do they offer stability to the "pseudoarthrosic" space.

Since the amount of antibiotic released is proportional to the surface area a "spacer" by its very surface configuration can offer only limited amount of antibiotic. In this context, injection moulded spacers is a misconceived concept. The glass-like surface of a mould injected ACAC spacer will only release antibiotic that is actually on the surface and that surface is reduced by the mould injection.

The second stage, of the two-stage revision, is carried out at a later date when infection is deemed to have been eradicated.

One or Two Stage Revision for Deep Infection?

Surgery of deep infection follows the basic principles: detailed debridement, closure of cavities and stabilization of the area. Two stage revisions aim to eliminate the infection before the arthroplasty is carried out at the second operation. It could be argued that if the first stage is unsuccessful, the second stage should not be carried out. If on the other hand the first stage is successful the second stage should not be necessary.

However, if one stage is considered as the first stage of a two stage operation then in over 80 % of cases the second stage would not be necessary. Each case must be treated according to the details: clinical radiographic, bacteriological.

The debate for one or two stage revision will no doubt continue. Resolution may come by force on economic rather than scientific evidence.

Early Indication of Outcome

Some indication of outcome of one-stage revision can be gained from very early clinical results. Freedom from pain is an excellent indicator and was found in 92 % of successful revisions. If the pain was relieved only partly some 48 % had a successful result. Persistence of pre-revision pain meant invariable failure – infection was not eradicated.

Quality of the bone stock for component fixation had no effect on the infection; success or failure was independent of bone quality found at revision. Long term mechanical outcome <u>was</u> dependent on the quality of bone; poor quality bone for component fixation increased the incidence of component loosening.

The conclusion must be: one-stage revision carried out early offers the best chance of success.

The problem is infection – the arthroplasty is incidental.

References

1. Wroblewski BM. One stage revision of infected cemented total hip arthroplasty. Clin Orthop Relat Res. 1986;211:103–7.
2. Raut VV, Siney PD, Wroblewski BM. One-stage revision of infected total hip replacements with discharging sinuses. J Bone Joint Surg Br. 1994;76-B:721–4.
3. Raut VV, Orth MS, Orth MC, Siney PD, Wroblewski BM. One stage revision arthroplasty of the hip for deep gram negative infection. Int Orthop. 1996;201:12–4.
4. Raut VV, Siney PD, Wroblewski BM. One-stage revision of total hip arthroplasty for deep infection. Long-term follow-up. Clin Orthop Relat Res. 1995;321:202–7.

Part III
Dislocation

Chapter 16
Dislocation

The fear of dislocation is undoubtedly the main reason why the small femoral head has not become universally popular (1978)

It was 15 years from the introduction of the operation and over 13,000 LFAs before Etienne, Cupic and Charnley [1] turned their attention to a detailed review of the incidence and causes of post-operative dislocation. The very low incidence was attributed to full exposure of the hip, preservation of the capsule, correct alignment of the components, secure re-attachment of the greater trochanter and the use of the abduction pillow post-operatively.

Monitoring of the results was routine. In an attempt to reduce the incidence of dislocation still further two changes were introduced: transverse reaming of the acetabulum and the change of the cup design to the long posterior wall (LPW) model. What was the clinical benefit of the changes? What was the effect on the already very low incidence of post-operative dislocation?

Transverse Reaming of the Acetabulum

Preparation of the acetabulum was a well defined sequence of steps; centering for the pilot hole, perforator then deepening and expanding reamers used alternatively. The acetabulum was reamed in cranial direction (Fig. 16.1).

The new cavity prepared matched the shape of the cup reasonably well and this allowed some degree of cement containment and pressurisation. With the cup placed more cranially, however, some limb shortening or at least inability to restore leg length, was probably inevitable, and was considered to be one factor that could contribute to post-operative dislocation. This was the technique until November 1970 when transverse reaming of the acetabulum was established. The detail of the technique was to use the same set of instruments but directing them transversely in line with anterior superior iliac spines (Fig. 16.2).

© Springer International Publishing Switzerland 2016

B.M. Wroblewski et al., *Charnley Low-Frictional Torque Arthroplasty of the Hip: Practice and Results*, DOI 10.1007/978-3-319-21320-0_16

Fig. 16.1 Reaming the
acetabulum in proximal
direction – guideline was
the patient's opposite
shoulder

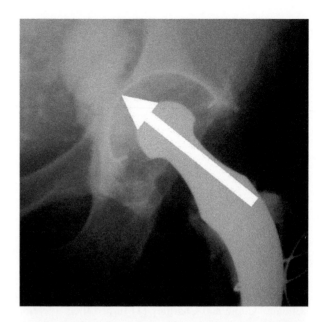

Fig. 16.2 Transverse
reaming of the
acetabulum – guideline
was the anterior superior
iliac spines

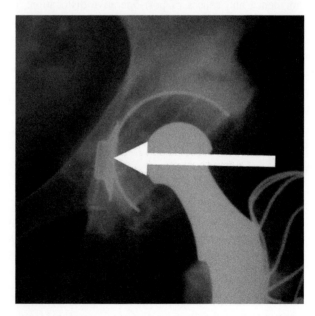

   The centering ring and the reamers had their lower margin at the level of the
"teardrop" the junction between the obturator foramen and the acetabulum. The
centre of rotation was thus brought distally, the cup could be placed at the more
anatomical level and thus contribute to leg length equalization.

Long Posterior Wall (LPW) Cup

The long posterior wall cup (LPW) (Fig. 16.3) was introduced in May 1972.

It was reasoned that the extension of the posterior wall of the cup, to the face of the hemisphere before the chamfer is machined, would allow a greater range of hip flexion and thus avoid dislocation even when the neck of the stem impinged on the anterior rim of the cup. Charnley was aware that the tendency; away from his Unit in Wrightington Hospital, was to antevert the cup. Anteverting the LPW cup would lead to impingement, posteriorly, and anterior dislocation. With the design went a warning: "*In accordance with previous teaching these sockets were inserted without anteversion.*"

The incidence of post-operative dislocation was studied over three consecutive periods. The results are summarised in Tables 16.1 and 16.2.

The very low dislocation rate is truly a remarkable record which continues to be questioned. Some explanation is essential.

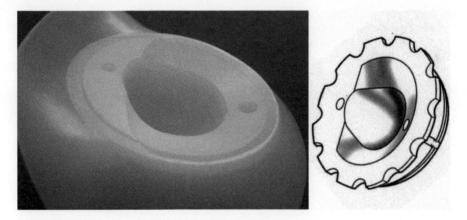

Fig. 16.3 The long posterior wall cup introduced in May 1972

Table 16.1 Incidence of post-operative dislocation 1966–1975

Period	Technique design	Number of LFAs	Number of dislocations	Dislocation %
1966/1969	Proximal reaming Standard cup	2825	25	0.9
Nov 1970 May 1972	Transverse reaming Standard cup	3495	18	0.5
1973/1975	Transverse reaming LPW cup	3495	13	0.4

Table 16.2 Recurrent dislocation and revision for dislocation

	Number of LFAs	Recurrent dislocation		Revision	
		No	%	No	%
Prior to 1971	3928	11	(0.3)	6	(0.2)
After 1971	4706	4	(0.08)	1	(0.02)

1971 data is excluded because of the overlap of both the technique of acetabular reaming and the introduction of the long posterior wall cup

Caution was the watchword in the early stages of the introduction of the operation into routine clinical practice. It was not unusual for patients to remain in hospital longer than the present routine; 2 or even 3 weeks was common.

- Early complications were recorded as part of the immediate post-operative care.
- Use of support – elbow crutches – for 3 months was the recommendation.
- Recording of complication at discharge was routine.
- Any complication noted after discharge or reported at follow-up was recorded on a separate pro-forma (as well as in the patients records), which were delivered to Charnley.
- Monitoring of complications in general and the individual surgeon's performance in particular, was maintained regularly.

Despite this routine it is probably inevitable that the complication remains underreported as episodes of subluxation have never been the subject of a publication. The same cannot be true of recurrent dislocation. Recurrent episodes undermine patient's confidence and bring the problem to the attention of the surgeon.

The review identified factors which were considered to contribute to postoperative dislocations.

Limb Shortening

The tear drop is used as the landmark. Higher than anatomical level of the cup was found in 50 % of dislocations but only in 16 % when the cup was placed at the anatomical level.

Stability

Instability of the arthroplasty, as determined at trial reduction, and before closure, was recorded in 21 % of dislocations but only 16.7 % when dislocation was not the complication.

Trochanteric Non-union

The results suggest, *"non-union of the greater trochanter would appear to be an important factor causing dislocation."*

It should come as no surprise that loss of abductor mechanism in general and trochanteric non-union in particular may play a role in dislocation after THA. The interpretation, however, may not be that simple. With the cup at the anatomical level the limb is lengthened. If the stem is placed in a valgus position, as was the practice before 1969 (though still advised in 1975), not only will the limb be lengthened further, but the stem may now encroach onto the trochanteric bed reducing the area of cancellous bed of the femur. The trochanter may have to be re-attached under tension, with the hip in an abducted position, increasing the likelihood of trochanteric non-union. Before 1971 trochanteric non-union was considered to be a contributory factor in 26 % of dislocations. After 1971 the incidence of post-operative dislocation was reduced, however, trochanteric non-union was the contributory factor in 33 %.

It is likely that the non-union of the greater trochanter should be viewed not as a radiographic finding but its effect on the hip stability. The separation of the trochanter need not result in dislocation if the abductors function, with the trochanteric fragment, as a "sesamoid". Hence, it is not merely non-union but the origin – insertion distance of the abductors – that is of interest.

Reference

1. Etienne A, Cupic Z, Charnley J. Post operative dislocation after Charnley low-friction arthroplasty. Clin Orthop Rel Res. 1979;1932:19–23.

Chapter 17
Revision for Recurrent or Irreducible Dislocation

Between November 1962 and June 1972, 14,672 LFAs had been carried out. Post-operative dislocation occurred in 92, an incidence of 0.63 % and included dislocation immediately after surgery reduced under the same general anaesthetic [1].

Twenty one, 0.14 % required revision. Three main causes were identified:

- Loss of abductor mechanism (trochanteric non-union),
- Shortening of the limb (high placement of the cup, low section of the femoral neck.
- Malorientation of components.

After the revision 16 patients (76.2 %) had no further dislocations, 1 had a single dislocation, while 4 (19 %) had more than one dislocation but managed to cope and did not require or want a further revision.

The review confirmed previously published information highlighting the essential points.

- Full exposure of the acetabulum,
- Correct preparation and placement of the cup at the correct level
- Neutral version of the cup with 45° angle open laterally.
- Correct level of femoral neck section.
- Stability of the joint at trial reduction.
- Secure re-attachment of the greater trochanter.

Comment

Dislocation of THA should not come as a surprise if it is considered that the natural and symptomatic joint is replaced by an artificial, neuropathic spacer. Absence of sensory input works both ways: freedom from pain but lack of warning of an

© Springer International Publishing Switzerland 2016

B.M. Wroblewski et al., *Charnley Low-Frictional Torque Arthroplasty of the Hip: Practice and Results*, DOI 10.1007/978-3-319-21320-0_17

impending dislocation – especially in the early post-operative period before healing of the deep soft tissues.

Recurrent dislocation undermines the patient's confidence and frustrates the surgeon who may seek refuge in alternative methods and designs. Exposures avoiding trochanteric osteotomy and use of larger diameter heads are intuitively considered to be likely immediate solutions. Both present new challenges but may appear more attractive than to follow what is a well established method in order to expand the understanding and improve on the results already achieved.

Revision for Dislocation Survivorship Analysis (Table 17.1 and Fig. 17.1)

Survivorship analysis [2, 3], with revision as the end-point, has become the accepted method of presenting follow-up results. In this method of analysis all operations are assigned to the same starting date.

Revision, a definite event, offers no information on any process leading up to it. It is essential that all findings at revision should be recorded. The number of findings will always be greater than the number of arthroplasties revised.

Early revisions, when the numbers are high, will have little effect on the overall pattern. With increasing follow-up as the number available for follow-up decline, each revision will have a more significant effect on that pattern. The method offers some indication on the pattern in relation to follow-up, but does not give the reasons for dislocation. The study of individual cases is essential. Furthermore, the method does not offer useful information if the number at the end-point is below 40 cases.

Table 17.1 Survivorship analysis: dislocation: end-point: revision for dislocation

Follow-up (years)	Number at start	Withdrawn	Failure	Number at risk	Cumulative Success rate	Confidence limits	
						Higher	Lower
0	22,066	0	0	22,066	100.0	100.0	100.0
1	22,066	5264	17	19,434	99.9	100.0	99.9
5	8092	1186	2	7499	99.8	99.9	99.7
10	3611	485	2	3368.5	99.6	99.8	99.4
15	1714	226	2	1601	99.2	99.6	98.8
20	817	136	0	749	98.9	99.6	98.1
25	318	67	0	284.5	98.5	99.9	97.1
30	71	21	0	60.5	98.0	100.0	94.5
35	11	4	0	9	98.0	100.0	89.0

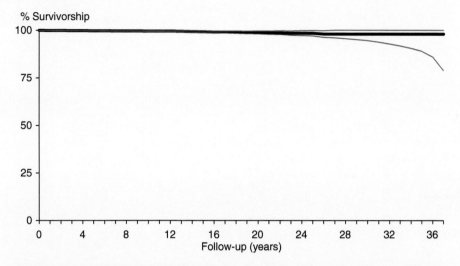

Fig. 17.1 Survivorship analysis – endpoint revision for dislocation or dislocation in combination with other findings – excluding infection

References

1. Fraser GA, Wroblewski BM. Revision of the Charnley low-friction arthroplasty for recurrent or irreducible dislocation. J Bone Joint Surg. (Br) 1981;63-B:552–5.
2. Kaplan EL, Meier P. Nonparametric estimation from incomplete observations. J Am State Assoc. 1958;53:457–81.
3. Lettin AF, Ware HS, Morris RW. Survivorship analysis and confidence intervals: an assessment with reference to the Stanmore total knee replacement. J Bone Joint Surg (Br). 1991;73-B: 729–31.

Chapter 18
Trochanteric Osteotomy and Dislocation

The operative procedure of total hip arthroplasty can be viewed as two separate but yet closely connected stages: the exposure of the joint and the fixation of the components.

Exposure by trochanteric osteotomy adds a further demand – the knowledge and understanding of osteotomy and osteosynthesis. Failure to achieve bony union, or any problems resulting from it, are immediately obvious. Benefits, if any, cannot be attributed to the method as they can only be assessed by the long-term results. Unfortunately, studies of long-term results, rarely, if ever, take into account the method of exposure as used at the primary operation. It is, therefore, not at all surprising that a combination of trochanteric osteotomy and 22.225 mm head diameter of the Charnley design strike fear into many orthopaedic surgeons. The net result is obvious – practice away from both the design and the method of exposure.

Evidence supporting this method of exposure will be found in the pages of this volume; arguments against should be looked up in various publications. Surgeons seriously committed to this method of treatment will have to consider the provision of revision facilities. This, now more extensive procedure, may demand more extensive exposures. It could be argued that trochanteric osteotomy could offer this, but revision procedure may not be the ideal time to undertake a new, to the surgeon, method of exposure. It is interesting that "extended trochanteric osteotomy" is gaining favour and even the length of the lateral femoral cortical fragment has become of sufficient interest to warrant a publication.

Trochanteric osteotomy is not merely the method that gives an excellent exposure of the acetabulum and the access to the medullary canal; it is an integral part of the concept. Medialisation of the cup with lateral and distal transposition of the greater trochanter, aimed to reduce the load on the hip, wear of the UHMWPE cup, protect the bone-cement interface and prolong the time during which the operation would remain successful. Charnley was well aware of the criticisms: broken wires, early dislocation, discomfort and "… *trochanteric non-union damaging the surgeon's reputation.*"

© Springer International Publishing Switzerland 2016   143
B.M. Wroblewski et al., *Charnley Low-Frictional Torque Arthroplasty of the Hip:
Practice and Results*, DOI 10.1007/978-3-319-21320-0_18

Charnley withheld the publication of the details of the technique until he "...
*believed that the problem of the trochanter has been truly solved or at least for ...
surgeons who were prepared to follow with understanding of the technique described."*

Using the "*cross-wire*" technique in 1020 LFAs, bony union was achieved in 95 %,
fibrous union in 2.6 % and complete trochanteric detachment in 2.4 %. The failure rate
was more common with residents in training than the senior staff but "... *relief of pain
was not significantly influenced by the defective trochanteric non-union."*

It is generally perceived that trochanteric osteotomy as the method of exposure when
combined with the 22.225 mm diameter head carries a high incidence of dislocation.

What are the facts?

Here we are concerned with the results spanning nearly 50 years of the clinical
practice of the Charnley LFA using trochanteric osteotomy and several methods of
reattachment usually using wires as the main material.

A review of 23,380 primary LFAs carried out over a 47 year period by over 350
surgeons at Wrightington Hospital is summarised in Tables 18.1, 18.2, 18.3, and 18.4.

The review does not take into account the seniority of the operating surgeon, or
the method of Trochanteric attachment.

Table 18.1 Primary LFA (1962 – 2009). Demographic details

Number of LFAs	23,380
Males	8271 (35.4 %)
Females	15,109 (64.6 %)
Age at LFA (years)	65 (12–95)
Follow-up years. Mean (range)	5.0 (0–40.5)

Note: Follow-up at zero years indicates revision for dislocation in the immediate post-operative period

Table 18.2 Primary LFA (1962 – 2009). Revision for/or with dislocation as operative finding

Trochanteric	Non-union	Union
Number (%)	1843 (7.9)	21,537 (92.1)
Dislocation No (%)	93 (5.1)	159 (0.74)
Revised No (%)	20 (1.1)	48 (0.22)
	68 (0.3)	

Table 18.3 Trochanteric osteotomy in primary LFA (1962–2009) and revision for or with dislocation. Gender difference

Gender	Male	Female
Number (%)	8271 (35.4)	15,109 (64.6)
Trochanteric non-union No (%) Revised No (%)	609 (7.4) 7 (1.1)	1234 (8.2) 13 (1.1)
Trochanteric union No (%) Revised No (%)	7662 (92.6) 12 (0.16)	13,875 (91.2) 36 (0.26)
Revised No (%)	19 (0.23)	49 (0.32)
	68 (0.3)	

Table 18.4 Trochanteric non-union and revision for dislocation: 20 revisions; (1.1 % of 1843 LFAs with non-union (0.09 % of the 23,380 LFAs))

20 revisions for dislocation	Time to revision: 5.2 years (0–14.5)
1st year:	5 revisions, 3 were for irreducible dislocation
2nd year:	3 revisions; one dislocation sustained in a heavy fall
3rd–9th year:	8 revisions: one loose stem
12th year onwards:	4 recurrent dislocations

Trochanteric Non-union and Revision for Dislocation

A detailed study of this group may offer some information concerning factors resulting in trochanteric non-union.

Trochanteric Union and Revision for Dislocation

Forty-eight revisions for dislocation: 0.2 % of the 21,537 with trochanteric union (and 0.18 % of the 23,380 LFAs). Mean time to revision was 13 years (0–27.5), 10 (20.8 %) in association with a loose cup.

– **35** revisions are the subject of detailed studies – of component position and orientation: None in this group had a loose cup or a loose stem
– **9** had a loose cup
– **1** had loose cup and stem
– **2** revisions with the UHMWPE cups fully worn out is an unusual occurrence as previously documented [1]. In these cases the cup remains firmly fixed medially
– **1** revision with a periprosthetic fracture of the femur.

Fears of a high incidence of revision for dislocation using trochanteric osteotomy and the 22.225 mm diameter head are unfounded [1]. Early problems are primarily technical and require understanding of the principle of osteosynthesis, attention to detail, training and practice. The skills acquired are essential if the individual undertakes this kind of surgery as a long-term commitment and not only to primary surgery.

The long term problem is wear and cup loosening and not one that can be attributed to either the concept or the design. Material issues are addressed in the appropriate section.

Summary

Out of 23,380 primary LFAs carried out over a 47-year period, 68 (0.3 %) had been revised for dislocation. In 14 of them (0.06 % of the whole group, 20.6 % of revisions for dislocation) contributing factors have been identified. In this context cup wear and loosening is the main, though very small, long-term problem. Here the low wear material combination and reduced diameter neck of the stem to put off impingement, would prove to be of benefit. The 35 revisions for dislocation with trochanteric union, 0.15 % of the whole series, will be subject to detailed studies.

The study and practice of methods of trochanteric osteotomy and reattachment would no doubt be of benefit accepting that revision surgery may be the inevitable consequence of long-term success in the very young patient.

Reference

1. Fraser GA, Wroblewski BM. Revision of the Charnley low-friction arthroplasty for recurrent or irreducible dislocation. J Bone Joint Surg (Br). 1981;63-B:552–5.

Chapter 19
Design of Components, Range of Movement. Impingement, Dislocation

There is little doubt that the dramatic occurrence of early post-operative dislocation undermines patient's confidence and disappoints the surgeon. Much has been written on the subject, many attempts have been made to analyse the factors involved and offer practical solutions. Most have focused on two aspects: diameter of the head of the femoral component and the orientation of the components in order to achieve the greatest range of movements with a minimum chance of neck-cup rim impingement.

It may, therefore, be of interest to consider some aspects of component design, range of movements, impingement and dislocation.

Hip Joint Movement

Movement, in space, can take place in three or a combination of the three planes. In a ball and socket articulation the range of movement is independent of the diameter of the ball. The movement in the natural hip joint is restricted to two planes; separation of articular surfaces does not occur naturally. The functional range is a combination of movement in two planes – rotation on the femoral neck is the combining motion. The range of rotation is independent of both the diameter of the head and the head-neck diameter ratio. Rotation shortens the hip capsule and resists separation of the joint spaces. In a design of any total hip arthroplasty the limit to the arc of movement is set by the contact of the neck of the stem with the rim of the cup.

© Springer International Publishing Switzerland 2016
B.M. Wroblewski et al., *Charnley Low-Frictional Torque Arthroplasty of the Hip: Practice and Results*, DOI 10.1007/978-3-319-21320-0_19

Head-Neck Diameter Ratio and Arc of Movement

In a design with a hemispherical cup, without a chamfer, a fully spherical head and
a neck of uniform diameter, the possible arc of movement, **is proportional to the
head-neck diameter (radius) ratio** (Fig. 19.1).

The arc of movement is given by the formula:-

$\theta = \cos^{-1}(^{r}/_{R})$ arc of movement
r = neck radius
R = head radius
∴ Full range of movement in a plane is $\theta \times 2$.

The arc of movement for head-neck diameter ratios up to 5:1 is given in Table 19.1
and Fig. 19.2. The relationship is not linear; when comparing ratios the resulting
scale is logarithmic. Increasing the head diameter and, therefore, the head-neck
ratio beyond 2.2:1 offers only moderate increase in the arc of movement.

Impingement

With the neck of the stem in a central position, with respect to the cup, impingement
will occur at one half of the possible arc of movement and may be conveniently
called "**the angle to impingement**". At that stage the summit of the head will be an
arc's distance (the arc based on the radius of the head) away from the cup rim
(Fig. 19.3). Movement past impingement will bring the summit of the head to the
rim of the cup reaching "**the limit of stability**" Movement past the limit of stability
will result in dislocation.

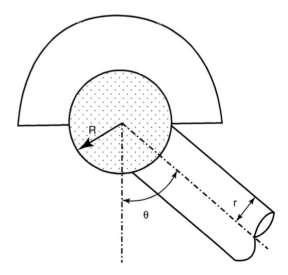

Fig. 19.1 Head-neck
diameter ratio and arc of
movement. One half of the
arc of movement (θ) in a
hemispherical cup: also
referred to as "angle to
impingement" – of the
neck of the stem on the rim
of the cup

Table 19.1 Head-neck diameter ratio and the possible arc of movement (10 mm diameter neck taken as probably the lowest limit acceptable)

Head – neck ratio	Range of movement (degrees)
1:1	0.0
1:2	67.1
1:4	88.8 natural hip
1:6	102.6
1:8	112.5
2:1	120.0
2:2	125.9 Charnley LFA
2:4	130.8
2:6	134.8
2:8	138.2
3:1	141.1
3:2	143.6
3:4	145.8
3:6	147.7
3:8	149.5
4:1	151.0
4:2	152.5
4:4	153.7
4:6	154.9
4:8	156.0
5:1	156.9

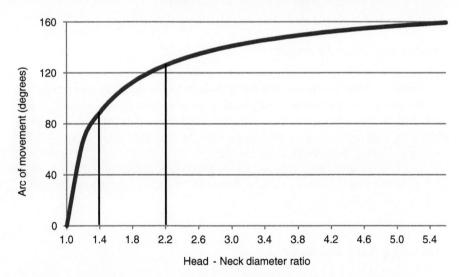

Fig. 19.2 Arc of movement, in a ball and socket articulation as an expression of head-neck diameter ratio. (Natural hip has a ratio of 1.4 degrees, Charnley hip has a ratio of 2.2 degrees)

Fig. 19.3 Angle to impingement and limit of stability. Summit of the head will be an arc's distance away from the cup rim

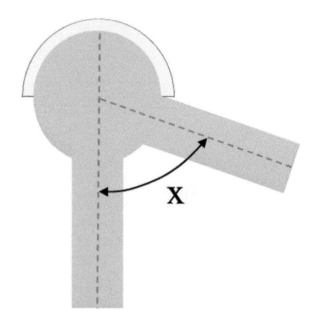

Increasing the Arc of Movements, Putting Off Impingement

There are four possible ways of achieving this objective.

Increasing Head Diameter

Conceptually attractive; in practice the limit is set by the size of the acetabular cavity. Increasing the diameter beyond a certain limit demands the use of hard on hard articulations and a departure from the clinically proven concept of low-frictional torque as well as the clinical experience with the materials: ultra high molecular weight polyethylene/metal/alumina ceramic.

Increasing head diameter may reduce the effective neck length. If the neck length is maintained then the offset would be increased. Reducing the thickness of the cup wall diminishes the usefulness of a chamfer.

Reducing Neck Diameter

A simple practical option; it increases the angle to impingement in proportion with the head-neck diameter (radius) ratio but reduces the angle to the limit of stability by the same degree.

Furthermore, since the strength of the neck is related to the cross-section area, reducing the neck diameter reduces its strength in the proportion of square of the radius. The material used becomes the limiting factor. In any symmetrical design, as

Fig. 19.4 Chamfer on cup. Fashioning the chamfer increases the angle to impingement but reduces the angle from impingement to the limit of stability by the same degree

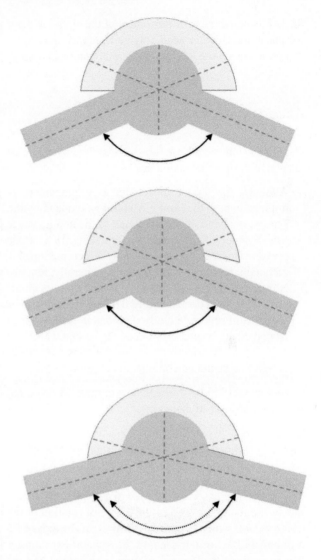

outlined here, there is no direct, straight line relationship, between the neck-head ratio and the possible arc of movement (Fig. 19.1) – the relationship is logarithmic (Fig. 19.2). This cannot be considered in hip resurfacing procedures.

Fashioning a Chamfer

A chamfer is produced by bevelling the edge of the rim of the cup. For ease of manufacture, inventory and surgical technique, the chamfer is usually circumferentially symmetrical. Fashioning the chamfer increases the angle to impingement but reduces the angle from impingement to the limit of stability by the same degree (Fig. 19.4).

Since functional range of movement of the hip joint is primarily anterior to the coronal plane, the chamfer need only be fashioned anteriorly. The examples that follow this principle are the long posterior wall cup of Charnley and the angle-bore cup.

Altering Cup Geometry

Cup dimensions may be reduced to less than a hemisphere. This, apparently simple change of design has its drawbacks.

– Although the arc of movement to impingement is increased, the arc from impingement to the limit of stability is reduced by the same angle.
– The external and the internal area of the cup is reduced in proportion of the cup rim – to – summit distance ($A = \pi\, r^2 h$) (Fig. 19.5). Reducing the area increases the pressure (load/unit area). This may affect fixation and increase wear.
– Although the angle of the cup, open laterally, remains unaltered, the head cover is reduced. To correct this the cup must be set more transversely to reduce the angle of the cup open laterally. The result may be reduced cup support within the acetabulum supero-laterally. This can be addressed either by deepening the acetabular cavity by encroaching on the medial wall, or by increasing the neck-shaft angle of the femoral component. This last adjustment is possible as a planned design of a stemmed component but not possible with resurfacing.

In a natural hip two further factors must be taken into account: the labrum and the offset: head-shaft distance.

The labrum, an extension of the acetabular rim increasing containment hence stability; being flexible does not offer a rigid restriction to movement.

The offset This anatomical configuration can be looked upon as evolutionary development imposed by the need of a single limb stance in bipedal gait. The offset moves the femur away from the centre of rotation of the head, increases the range of hip **flexion which is mainly rotation on the axis of the neck**. Quadruped hip has a minimal offset or neck length. Movement is primarily limited to saggital plane. The anatomy of the femoral articulation is more like a saddle than a ball and socket.

Impingement and Bone-Implant Interface

– Freedom of movement at the articulation is related to the design.
– Resistance to movement at the bone-implant interface is proportional to the surface area in contact, the method to achieve this and maintain long term.

Impingement and Bone-Implant Interface					153

Fig. 19.5 Reducing cup
dimensions: The external
and the internal area of the
cup is reduced in
proportion of the cup
rim – to – summit distance
$(A = \pi\, r^2 h)$

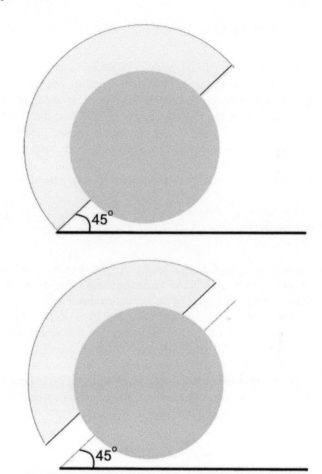

In order to enhance the ease of motion at the articulation, while resisting movement at bone-implant interface, the largest possible radii difference between the head and the outer cup margin should be employed (Fig. 19.1).

At impingement the mechanics of the articulation change significantly. The lever of rotation, hitherto the radius of the head, is extended to the point of impingement of the neck on the rim of the cup and becomes slightly greater than the diameter of the head. This increases the turning moment at the bone-implant interface. The area of contact between the head and the cup is reduced increasing the load. The displacement of the head out of the cup results in stretching of the capsule. The displaced volume is proportional to the head diameter. Thus, the greater the head, the more extensive is the damage to soft tissues and greater the resulting laxity [1]. Single episodes of impingement may not be a problem, repeated episodes threaten the integrity of the bone-cement interface and may, in time, result in increased wear and cup loosening.

Practical Approach

In clinical practice decisions must be made, based on all the information available, and then put into practice. The issue becomes ever more complex when hip joint exposure, availability of suitable bone-stock, preparation of bone and cup positioning and the method of fixation are taken into account. Added to this is the stem with the range of possible modular head sizes and functional neck dimensions. All this is carried out in an attempt to recreate a near normal anatomically and mechanically arrangement while avoiding impingement and ensuring stability. **The greater the modularity of the system the later the decision is likely to be made**.

Examination of Explanted Components

Pursuing the line of design, head size, neck diameter and impingement and possibility of dislocation in THA, we examined 13 sets of explanted hip components of various designs (subject of further detailed studies).

The head diameter ranged from 22.225 to 46 mm. In only eight was the head-neck diameter ratio 2:1. In the remaining five it was less despite the head sizes greater than 22.225 mm. If the cup wall thickness of 10 mm is considered desirable, then the outer UHMWPE cup diameter should have been at least 45–66 mm – probably beyond the available bone stock in a fair proportion of cases (The Charnley 22.225 mm diameter head with a 10 mm diameter neck was not in this collection although the 12.5 mm diameter neck was).

Natural Hip Joints

Examination of examples of proximal femora clearly shows the variation of both the head and the neck dimensions and whether the measurement of the neck is taken in the coronal or saggital plane.

The head-neck diameter ratio was found to be in the range of 1.3:1 and 1.8:1.

Assuming a hemispherical acetabulum the possible range of movement, in a plane, would be 50–77° and reorientation of the acetabulum would not increase that range. Since in a natural hip this range of movement is greater and orientation of the acetabulum would not alter that range, what is the explanation? We need to consider only the motion anterior to the coronal plane; other movements, excluding rotation, do not reach the 77° maximum.

The "thigh – chest" position can only be achieved either with the acetabulum "deficient" anteriorly, flexion of the spine, rotation on the neck of the femur or the combination of all three.

It becomes clear that with a head-neck ratio of a natural hip, the acetabulum cannot be either hemispherical or orientated in a position as to improve

that ratio and, therefore, the range of movement. The natural acetabulum must be asymmetrical both in structure and function with freedom of flexion combined with adduction and internal rotation with stability posteriorly.

Since the acetabulum is asymmetrical it cannot be viewed as being anti – or -retroverted. The variable is the extent of the asymmetry – the relationship between the anterior and the posterior acetabular rims – and not change in the position of the acetabulum as a whole.

<u>Note</u> When considering the range of movements of the hip joint what is commonly omitted is the rotation on the axis of the neck; combined with the offset it offers greater range that is often commonly considered. "Flexion" of the hip is in fact rotation on the neck of the femur, to a large degree!

Practical Application and Clinical Experience

Theoretical considerations highlight the complexity of the geometry of the ball and socket articulation of the normal hip joint and even more so its role in the function and stability of the total hip arthroplasty.

The question posed must be: does the head size play any role in the incidence of dislocation after primary total hip arthroplasty?

The Charnley LFA is the concept with the longest clinical experience. It continues to be under the most severe scrutiny because of the 22.225 mm diameter head. It may, therefore, be of interest to review the incidence of revisions for dislocation after primary Charnley LFA.

Reduced Diameter (10 mm) Neck of the Charnley Stem and Post-Operative Dislocation After Primary Low-Frictional Torque Arthroplasty

In the development of his hip replacement Charnley pursued the principle of low-frictional torque. To achieve this aim the diameter of the head of the femoral component was reduced, in stages, from $1^5/_8$ in. (41.5 mm) to $^7/_8$ in. (22.225 mm) [2].

Post-operative dislocation with the 22.225 mm diameter head has not been a problem in primary operations: the reported incidence was 0.4–0.8 % [3, 4].

Fear of post-operative dislocation continues to be an argument used by the advocates of large diameter heads [5, 6].

Reducing the diameter of the neck of the Charnley stem from 12.5 to 10 mm increases the range of movement in a plane from 90 to 108° [7] before impingement, and increases the head-neck ratio from 1.78:1 to 2.22:1. Charnley suggested the modification in June 1982. This was made possible by the introduction of high nitrogen content stainless steel and the cold-forming process in the stem manufacture resulting in a much stronger material ORTRON (DePuy International, Leeds, U.K.).

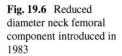

Fig. 19.6 Reduced diameter neck femoral component introduced in 1983

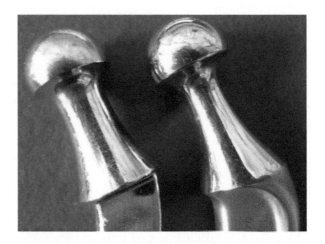

Did reducing the diameter of the neck of the Charnley stem (from 12.5 to 10 mm) offer further benefit in reducing the low incidence of dislocation after primary Charnley low-frictional torque arthroplasty (LFA) (Since the benefit of the reduced diameter neck on the incidence of cup loosening was anticipated on a theoretical basis [7] and confirmed in clinical practice [8] the design has become a standard item; we did not consider that a randomized study would be justified.).

The reduced diameter 10 mm neck Charnley stem (Fig. 19.6) was introduced into routine clinical practice in October 1983 after testing to the then DD91 British Standards Institution criteria [9].

Our database over the period from November 1962 to January 2005 was reviewed selecting primary LFAs and identifying cases of post-operative dislocations; occurring within the first year after the operation, after the first year, and revisions for dislocation. We excluded two groups of cases: those with stems which had shorter than standard neck lengths: three quarter length, CDH and mini stems and also "offset-bore" cups [10] as they did not have a chamfer. All the operations were carried out in the Charnley-Howorth clean air enclosure with lateral trans-trochanteric approach by over 300 surgeons.

During the 42-year period 22,300 primary LFAs had been carried out. In 14,051 a standard neck diameter of 12.5 mm was used and in 8247 hips (from October 1983), a reduced 10 mm neck diameter was used. The detailed results are shown in Table 19.2.

Reducing the diameter of the neck of the Charnley stem from 12.5 to 10 mm and thus increasing the range of movement by 18° did not have a statistically significant effect on the already low incidence of post-operative dislocation or revisions for dislocation.

Our findings indicate that with the Charnley design and the surgical technique the 90–108° range of movements caters for the vast majority of activities.

Impingement is an unlikely cause of dislocation unless through malposition of components [4, 5] or gross anteversion of the cup using the posterior approach [11].

Table 19.2 Incidence of, and revision for, dislocation after primary Charnley LFA with standard 12.5 mm, and reduced 10 mm diameter neck stem

	Standard (12.5 mm) diameter neck	Reduced (10 mm) diameter neck
Number of LFAs	14,051	8247
Male	4611	3179
Female	9440	5068
Age: years	65.3 (12–91)	63.7 (13–93)
Follow-up: years	4.8 (0–38)	4.4 (0–22)
Dislocation		
Early	111 (0.79 %)	73 (0.88 %)
Late	205 (1.46 %)	100 (1.21 %)
Revision	41 (0.29 %)	21 (0.25 %)

N.B. Zero follow-up denotes death within the first post-operative year

Impingement [7] is considered to be the main cause of the linear incidence of aseptic cup loosening with the increasing depth of cup penetration [12, 13]. The long term benefit of the reduced, 10 mm, diameter neck Charnley stem is in the reduction of the incidence of aseptic cup loosening equivalent to 2 mm of cup penetration [8].

Angle Bore Cup

The angle bore cup design was conceived and introduced into clinical practice in an attempt to address post-operative dislocation in revisions of failed total hip arthroplasties.

It simulates the asymmetry of both the structure, as well as the function, of the natural acetabulum. The asymmetry of the natural acetabulum is normally referred to as anteversion.

The terminology in common use implies that the natural acetabulum is symmetrical in structure, but variable in orientation, with respect to the pelvis. This is not so. The natural acetabulum allows full range of movements anterior to the coronal plane while ensuring stability – posteriorly to that plane. The angle-bore cup design matches this asymmetry.

In the manufacture of the component, the centre of the hemisphere of the plastic is approached at 45° from the antero-inferior direction, thus creating the chamfer anteriorly and inferiorly allowing freedom of flexion, adduction and internal rotation. The angle and the direction of the bore creates a recess postero-superiorly, simulating the labrum, offering stability (Fig. 19.7). The component is side-specific.

It must not be anteverted!

In 1039 revisions of failed total hip arthroplasties, at a mean follow-up of 9 years (0–20.6), the incidence of re-revisions for dislocation was 2.1 %.

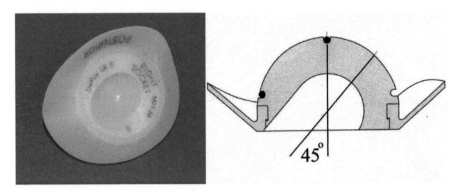

Fig. 19.7 Angle-bore cup. The angle of the bore is at 45°

In 65 revisions for dislocation the success rate was 89.2 % after first revision, and 96.9 % after second revision [14].

References

1. Charnley J. Low friction arthroplasty of the hip. Theory and practice. Berlin: Springer-Verlag; 1979. p. 13.
2. Charnley J. Arthroplasty of the hip. A new operation. Lancet 1961;1(7187):1129–37.
3. Etienne A, Cupic Z, Charnley J. Post-operative dislocation after Charnley low-friction arthroplasty. Clin Orthop. 1978;132:19–23.
4. Frazer GA, Wroblewski BM. Revision of Charnley low-friction arthroplasty for recurrent or irreducible dislocation. J Bone Joint Surg (Br). 1981;63-B:552–5.
5. Bartz RL, Noble PC, Kakadia NR, Tullos HS. The effect of femoral component head size on posterior dislocation after the artificial hip joint replacement. J Bone Joint Surg Am. 2000;82-A:1300.
6. Berry JD, von Koch M, Schleck CD, Harmesen WS. Effect of femoral head diameter and the operative approach on risk of dislocation after primary total hip arthroplasty. J Bone Joint Surg Am. 2005;82-A:245.
7. Wroblewski BM. Direction and rate of socket wear in Charnley low-friction arthroplasty. J Bone Joint Surg (Br). 1985;67-B:757–61.
8. Wroblewski BM, Siney PD, Fleming PA. Reduced diameter neck and its effect on the incidence of cup loosening in the Charnley LFA. J Bone Joint Surg (Br). 2005;87-B:43.
9. British Standards Institution Method of determination of endurance properties of stemmed femoral components of hip joint prostheses. DD91 1984 (Amendment 4876).
10. Izquierdo-Avino RJ, Siney PD, Wroblewski BM. Polyethylene wear in the Charnley offset bore acetabular cup. A radiological analysis. J Bone Joint Surg (Br). 1996;78-B:82–4.
11. Porter P, Stone MH. Total hip arthroplasty using the Wroblewski golf-ball cup inserted through the posterior approach. A high rate of dislocation. J Bone Joint Surg (Br). 2004;86-B:643–7.
12. Wroblewski BM. Charnley low friction arthroplasty in patients under the age of 40 years. In: Sevastik, Goldie I, editors. The young patient with degenerative hip disease. Stockholm: Almquist & Wiksell International; 1985. p. 197–201.
13. Wroblewski BM, Siney PD, Fleming PA. Charnley low frictional torque arthroplasty in patients under the age of 51 years. J Bone Joint Surg (Br). 2002;84-B:540–3.
14. Wroblewski BM, Siney PD, Fleming PA. The angle bore acetabular component and dislocation after revision of a failed total hip replacement. J Bone Joint Surg (Br). 2006;88-B:184–7.

Part IV
Stem

Chapter 20
Stem Design and Fixation

Stem design and its use in total hip arthroplasty have evolved from treatment of fractures of the neck of the femur. Limited exposure in an elderly frail patient, failure to achieve fracture reduction or fixation, demanded a more definitive treatment – a hemiarthroplasty. The exposure was adequate for the purpose; the acetabulum was not exposed; femoral head served to gauge the size. Access to the medullary canal was limited through the neck of the femur, merely for the insertion of the hemiarthroplasty. Cement was not used.

Addition of acrylic cement for stem fixation was considered merely a minor aspect of the procedure. It was at this stage that complications, attributed to the use of acrylic cement, were published. The explanation, in retrospect, is obvious – large medullary canal, fatty marrow, cement trapping air and fat, stem acting as a piston injecting the medullary contents into the patient's circulation. With the increasing understanding of the function of the stem in the mechanics of total hip arthroplasty the emphasis changed from "replacement" to "reconstruction" of hip mechanics. Exposure demanded a better view of the acetabulum and the access to the medullary canal, not through the neck of the femur, but through the piriform fossa. Longer follow-up, in patients with osteoarthritis, revealed new problems. Stem loosening and fracture were the new complications. They served as a source of information for further developments. It is probably correct to suggest that it was the stem fracture, "an event": rather than the stem loosening, "a process": that has made a bigger contribution to our understanding of the function of the stem. This has led to the changes of stem design, materials, methods of manufacture, and the technique of stem fixation.

Stem Design

Stem design and the method of fixation are better understood if an attempt is made to answer the basic question: What is the rationale dictating the use of a stemmed femoral component? It serves, primarily, as an anchorage and support for the

© Springer International Publishing Switzerland 2016
B.M. Wroblewski et al., *Charnley Low-Frictional Torque Arthroplasty of the Hip: Practice and Results*, DOI 10.1007/978-3-319-21320-0_20

extra-medullary portion of the stem. In its proximal part it must resist torsion, in its distal part it must prevent tilting. A stemmed femoral component can be best considered as having three parts, the head, the neck and the shaft. Each one serves a different function and may, therefore, be subject to variations in materials and design, yet together they form an integral part both of the stem and of the arthroplasty.

The Head

The two parameters are the size and the materials used.

The size would be related to the frictional torque of the design, the perceived concept of stability and wear characteristics of the materials used. The materials would be related primarily to strength, wear and the ultimate fate of wear products within the body environment. In any modular system the head-neck assembly would have to be considered.

The Neck

The dimensions of interest are: strength and diameter; hence head-neck ratio and therefore the range of movements, in a plane, before impingement; the neck length and therefore its contribution to limb length; and the neck-shaft angle which would determine the offset of a particular design.

The Shaft

It is the understanding of the function of the intramedullary portion, in the function of the arthroplasty as a whole, that is the essential aspect both in the stem design and the methods of stem fixation.

Stem Design and Methods of Fixation

The Shaft

The intramedullary part serves primarily as an anchorage and a support for the extramedullary part: the head and the neck. In clinical practice two methods are used to achieve that objective: a single stem-femur complex "interference fit" or male/female tapers engaging under load "taper fit".

Interference Fit: A Single Stem-Femur Complex

The aim, both of the stem design and the surgical technique, is to achieve an integral stem-femur unit. To increase the surface area of the stem-bone contact, the surface of the stem is bead or porous coated. To encourage bony on-growth/in-growth the surface is treated; as in hydroxyapatite designs.

The instrumentation and the surgical technique are aimed at achieving an interference fit between the implant and the endosteum. The final step, in stem fixation at surgery, is a combination of rasp effect of the advancing stem, interference-fit, elasticity of the femur, strain generation and relaxation. The immediate fixation is a combination of interference fit and the elasticity of the femur. The quality of that fixation is governed by "the last hammer blow" and is determined by the contact at the asperities. The long-term anticipated quality of fixation is by bony on-growth or in-growth – osseointegration. Osseointegration is the characteristic of the skeleton. Thus the implant is controlled by the designer and the manufacturer, while the ultimate mode of fixation – osseointegration is "under the control" of the patient's skeleton. Surgical technique now plays a minor role and is largely replaced by the implant – a commodity that can be sold at a profit.

The advantage is an undemanding simplicity. The disadvantage of the method is the inability to judge the quality of fixation at surgery – hence fractures of the femur, at surgery, may result. If osseointegration is achieved the problems of stem extraction, at revision, will have to be addressed.

Taper Fit: Male and Female Tapers Engaging Under Load

The method takes the advantage of the long established engineering principle the male and female tapers engaging under load. When the system becomes load-bearing it must allow a slip of the male taper, the stem, within the female taper, the cement.

The Male Taper: The Stem

For the stem to be allowed to slip within the cement mantle, it must have a polished surface, continuous taper, it must not be supported distally.

The Female Taper: The Cement

The cement must be of good quality and well supported by strong cancellous bone over the largest possible area.

Surgical Technique

The surgical technique is the essential element of the method.

The objective is to offer the largest possible area of contact between cement and bone and thus reduce pressure per unit area and to ensure the strongest possible bone-cement interface in order to resist both hoop and torsional loads while avoiding proximal strain shielding of the femur. It must also allow a limited slip of the stem within the cement mantle.

The method is highly design and technique dependant. Stem design can no longer be a replacement for the surgical technique, and the technique is not a commodity that can be sold at a profit.

It cannot, therefore, come as a surprise that in clinical practice there is a move away from the demanding surgical technique towards the "more forgiving" implants, as well as "cementless" fixation of components. (A "forgiving" implant is a rather unfortunate term; it admits transgression without promise of repentance.) "Cementless" fixation on the other hand does not define a method of fixation except by stating what it is not. An addition of "porous" or "HA" coating merely describes the surface finish of the implant and not the method of fixation.

Stem Design: The Taper

The geometry of the medullary canal presents a range of shapes and dimensions. They may be graphically and unconventionally described by the capital letters U, V, Y (Figs. 20.1, 20.2, and 20.3). (Though clearly this can only be a rough scheme and any variation will demand a combination of the letters; an interesting but not a particularly helpful exercise). The surgery of total hip arthroplasty demands a tapered stem irrespective of these variations. It is here that the benefit of the acrylic cement becomes so obvious. It can provide of the whole range of "custom built" individually intimate shapes and sizes with the largest possible contact area, while the stem can now be considered as a separate entity within the cement mantle – a taper fit. (No such contact is possible with a simple interference, "cementless", fit). Although the concept is one of a simple wedge, the dimensions of the medullary canal and the function of the hip demand a more complex design – a wedge with an offset.

The Taper

The taper must allow a predictable, limited slip of the stem within the cement. The stem must also be bulky enough to resist torsion and its effects; loosening and fracture and also allow transfer of the load to the most proximal part of the femur. The dimensions of the taper are primarily governed by the length of the shaft of the stem.

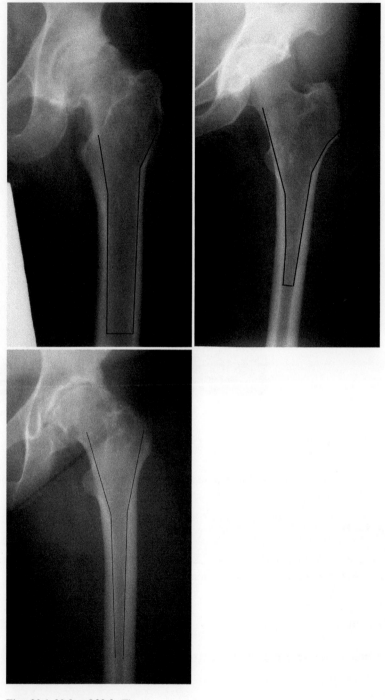

Figs. 20.1, 20.2 and 20.3 The geometry of the medullary canal presented graphically and unconventionally described by the capital letters U, V, Y

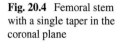

Fig. 20.4 Femoral stem with a single taper in the coronal plane

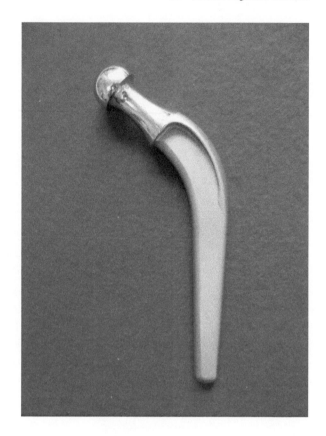

Taper Geometry

Three configurations are possible: single, double or triple, proximal to distal taper.

Single Taper

Taper in the coronal plane (Fig. 20.4). Excellent in resisting torsion but the overall bulk of the stem is governed by the dimensions of the medullary canal.

Double Taper

Tapers both in the coronal plane and the saggital planes (Fig. 20.5).

Fig. 20.5 Femoral stem
with a double taper. Tapers
both in the coronal plane
and the saggital planes

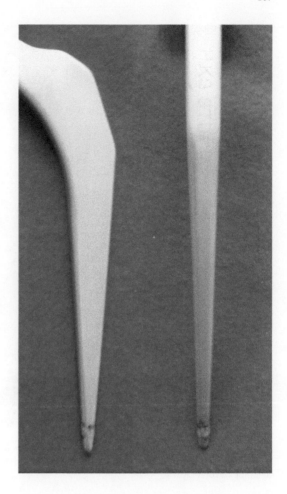

Triple Taper

Design takes the advantage of greater dimensions of the proximal medullary canal
by adding to the bulk of the stem – laterally – thus forming the third lateral to medial
taper (Fig. 20.6).

The third taper is continuous throughout the whole length of the shaft of the
stem, resists torsion more efficiently and transfers the load over a greater area of
cement and the proximal femur.

Stem Length

The length of the stem shaft is dictated by its resistance to tilting, the bulk to its
resistance to torsion and fracture, while the tapers to cater for the two within the
confines of the medullary canal. The result is inevitably a compromise; mechanically

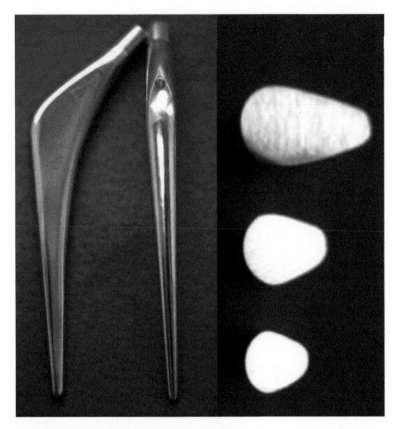

Fig. 20.6 Femoral stem with a Triple Taper design takes the advantage of greater dimensions of the proximal medullary canal by adding to the bulk of the stem – laterally – thus forming the third lateral to medial taper

sound and aesthetically pleasing to the eye. In theory, no shorter that 10 cm, in practice variable, to counterbalance the length of the extramedullary portion – the neck and the head; in practical terms "as long as necessary but as short as possible".

Surface Finish

If the principle of slip of the stem within the cement mantle is accepted, then surface finish must be polished to allow that slip.

Stem Offset

By convention, the stem offset is measured by the distance from the centre of rotation of the head of the femoral component and the line drawn through the centre of the shaft of the stem, the two lines joined at a right angle, the distance measured in

Fig. 20.7 Conventional
method of measuring stem
offset A (Reproduced from
Wroblewski [1])

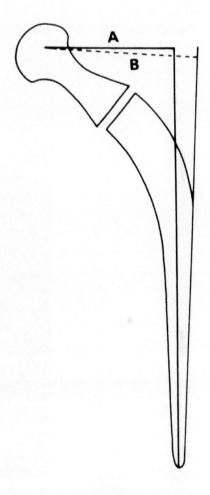

millimetres (Fig. 20.7). Although simple and unambiguous its application in clinical practice may be less so. A stem that has no obvious straight section, a curved stem, is one such an example. Also stem fracture originates, usually, on the antero-lateral aspect of the stem, it could be argued that the offset distance should be measured from the lateral border and not the centre of the stem.

Placement of the stem at surgery will also have an effect on the **functional offset** of the femur-stem complex. A central position of the stem within the medullary canal can be accepted as fulfilling the offset definition criteria. A valgus position will reduce the functional offset bringing the shaft of the femur closer to the pelvis thus reducing the abductor level and increasing the load on the hip. The expected consequence will be increasing wear rate of the cup and, therefore, a higher incidence of cup loosening. The position of the stem will also have an effect on the distribution of the cement and the behaviour of the stem (Fig. 20.8). A valgus stem position is more likely to separate the cement mantle (as seen on the A–P radiograph) into medial proximal layer and the distal lateral layer – the stem now allowed an unrestrained slip between the two layers of cement. Varus placement of the stem will have the same effect.

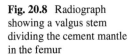

Fig. 20.8 Radiograph showing a valgus stem dividing the cement mantle in the femur

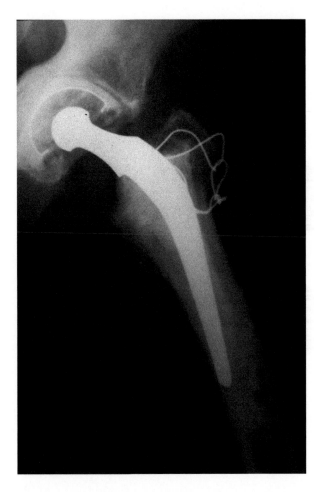

Accessing the medullary canal, through the sectioned neck of the femur, will direct the stem posteriorly. This stem position has been the commonest error observed in clinical practice at revision (Fig. 20.9).

Surgical Technique

The practical application of a concept into a mechanically demanding operative technique in order to achieve long-term success. It demands the understanding of the concept of the design, the details of the surgical technique and the effects of patient's activities. The objective; not only as an immediate technical performance, but as a long-term successful result. Adequate exposure to gain unimpeded access to the medullary canal, removal of poor quality cancellous bone and clearing the marrow spaces of blood and fat, the handling of cement from the time of mixing to delivering, pressurisation at stem insertion – each aspect must be understood and well rehearsed.

Fig. 20.9 Radiograph showing a lateral view of the femur (Note the distribution of cement mantle). The stem has been placed front to back, proximal to distal

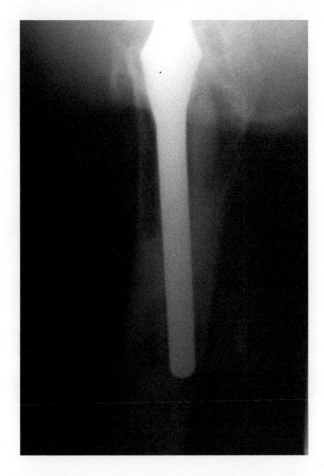

Two further details must be taken into account: resistance to torsion and distal stem support. Resistance to torsion, proximally, will be improved by adequate stem support postero-medially. It is here that the role of the anatomical calcar, calcar femorale, is significant.

Calcar Femorale

In the development of the proximal femur the lesser trochanter is formed by traction of the ilio-psoas which separates the medial femoral cortex into two layers – the outer cortex and the inner thin sheet of cortical bone postero-medially, the calcar femorale (Fig. 20.10). The two join postero-medially to form the thick medial femoral neck popularly but erroneously referred to as "calcar". With advancing age and declining function the bone which is "furthest away from function" is gradually resorbed (Wolff's Law). It is this process that is responsible for the thinning of bone cortices and the apparent expansion of the medullary canal. Thinning and loss of

Fig. 20.10 Calcar
Femorale (*arrow*)

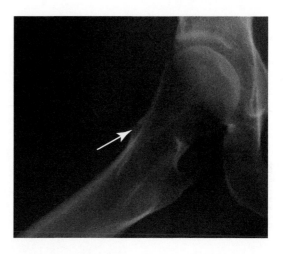

calcar femorale is a part of that process. In the normal hip the result is loss of the
support for the head of the femur and femoral neck fracture with the postero-medial
comminution.

If the calcar is not cleared and the stem is placed centrally – in both planes – then
the proximal part of the stem will be opposed to the calcar femorale – without supporting layer of cement (Figs. 20.10 and 25.4).

It is essential that calcar be cleared to good quality cancellous bone before injecting cement.

Distal Stem Support

If the taper fit is part of both the stem design and the surgical technique, then it must
be accepted that distal stem support is contraindicated. Proximal load transfer – the
objective of the triple taper design – cannot be achieved if a stem is distally supported
(Figs. 20.11, 20.12, and 20.13). In practice the intramedullary bone block technique,
with the tip of the stem penetrating into the cancellous bone of the bone block, thus
avoiding distal stem support. Component fixation is the single most important aspect
of this type of operation. Using cement is entirely within the surgeon's control.

A Combination of Concepts

Stem designs and finer details of surgical technique have evolved with clinical
experience.

Fig. 20.11 Radiograph of
a secure femoral stem
showing fracture tip of
cement

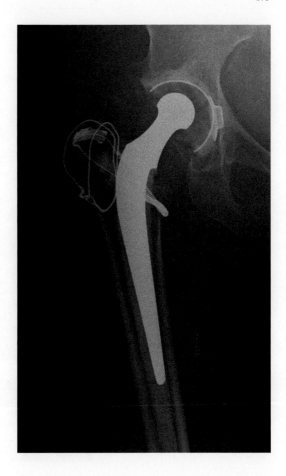

Flanged Stem

*The dorsal flange is intended to make the upper levels of cement function more effectively
in load transmission, thereby reducing the amount of stress reaching down to the mid-level
of the stem where fatigue fractures are prone to develop. This feature makes what at the
moment is an imponderable contribution to the strength in the in-vivo situation* (Fig 20.14)

Further comments on the evolution of the design and the clinical results is highlighted in the relevant section of this work.

Stem Precoat

The surface of the stem is covered with a layer of acrylic cement in order to form an
integral complex. The objective is, presumably, to provide secure fixation between
the precoated stem and the medullary cement. If so the concept is flawed. If the
precoat-cement interface remains intact, as intended by the design, decoupling

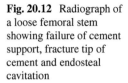

Fig. 20.12 Radiograph of
a loose femoral stem
showing failure of cement
support, fracture tip of
cement and endosteal
cavitation

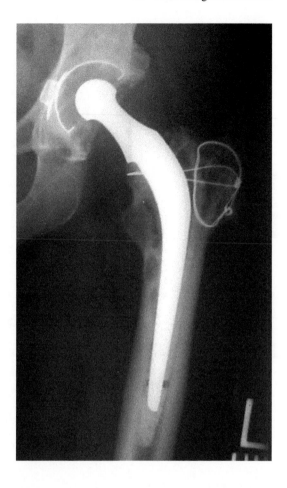

between cement and stem is not possible then any movement can only occur at the
cement-bone interface. If the precoat-stem interface fails then the cement is exposed
to the rough surface of the stem. None of the two offer the safety of taper-fit.

Matt Surface Finish of the Stem Used with Cement

Although it may be viewed differently now, this combination, certainly with the
Charnley stem, was an attempt to work-harden the surface layer and ablate any irregu-
larities that could possibly have acted as stress risers and be the cause of stem fracture.
The method of surface treatment became refined but the matt appearance remained.

Calcar-Collar Contact: Or (Collar-Medial Femoral Neck Contact)

It is probably correct to suggest that in clinical practice two designs have emerged:
"accidental" and "deliberate".

Fig. 20.13 Radiograph of
a fractured femoral stem,
showing failure of cement
support and fracture tip of
cement

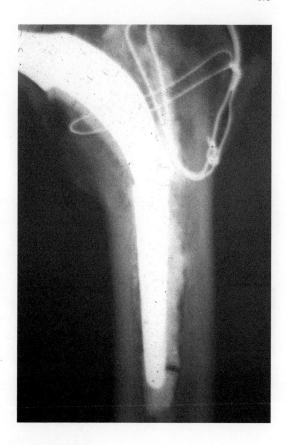

Accidental Calcar-Collar Contact Design (Fig. 20.15)

The Charnley original "flat-back" and "round-back" fit into this category. The reason rather than a rationale is easy to understand. The stem was machined from a solid bar. The head and the neck, down to its base, is the result of circular motion on a lathe while the shaft is machined on a flat. (Initially stems were machined from the uniform length blank. The interesting side issue, not readily appreciated, was that as the neck of the prosthesis was made shorter as in the three-quarter neck, mini or the CDH stem, the shaft of the stem became proportionally longer!). The "collar" was not designed for its function, but was a by-product of the method of stem manufacture. In clinical practice, however, it served a very useful purpose; the end point for stem insertion at surgery.

Deliberate Calcar-Collar Contact Design (Fig. 20.16)

The origin of this design is probably a continuation of the Moore and Thompson hemiarthroplasty as used originally. The support for the stem was the base of the neck resting on the sectioned femoral neck, the collar was truly load bearing.

Fig. 20.14 Charnley
flanged stem – final
version 1982

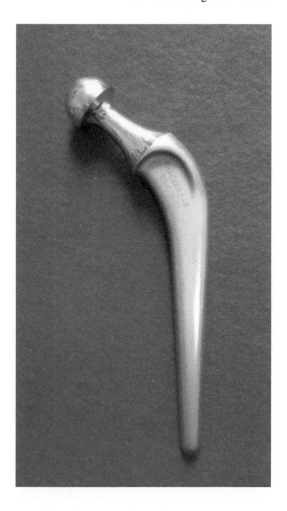

Extension of this principle to cemented total hip arthroplasty may appear to be logical and reasonable. There are, however, limitations which must be taken into account:

- Since the femoral neck is anteverted the collar of the stem must either be designed
  accordingly, demanding a right and left stem, or the stem anteverted, to a varying
  degree, deliberately at operation.
- The angle of the section of the neck must be made in a fashion so that the collar
  must fit accurately. Simple instrumentation would achieve this.
- Variety of femoral sizes and offsets demands a range of collar/stem
  configurations.
- The collar must come to rest and remain on the sectioned medial femoral neck
  the "calcar".
- If the stem fails to slip within the cement mantle or the "calcar" below the collar
  becomes resorbed, then the collar would serve no useful purpose other than contribute to a "non-return valve" effect and endosteal cavitation below the collar.

Fig. 20.15 Radiograph of
a collared femoral stem
showing "Accidental"
"calcar" collar contact

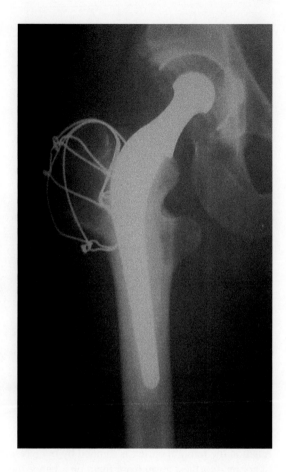

- Since the load on the hip during activity is from the antero-superior direction, the net effect is postero-medial deflection of the proximal part of the stem, the collar would be in shear and not in compression.
- The collar may act as a hinge and contribute to stem fracture [1] (Fig. 20.17).

There are too many uncertainties for the concept to function consistently in clinical practice.

Bone Responds to Function

If we accept that bone responds to function (Wolff) then we must accept that the introduction of stemmed femoral components will have an effect on mode of load transfer. In a natural hip the load is transferred across the acetabulum to the cortico-cancellous bone of the head and neck of the femur then to the femoral cortex. Medullary canal does not take part in load transfer. With advancing age and declining

Fig. 20.16 Radiograph of
a collared femoral stem
showing "Calcar" – collar
contact by design. The
design and the technique
did not prove sufficiently
beneficial to be routinely
used

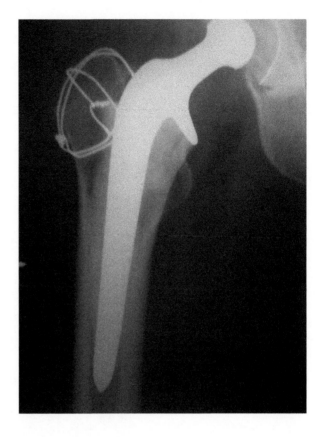

function the femoral cortex is thinned by bone resorption from the innermost layers
of cortex – furthest away from function – hence the expanding medullary canal.

The introduction of stemmed prosthesis alters the pattern of load transfer – the
medullary canal now becomes load bearing, at least partly, and certainly more
distally than in a natural hip. Proximal strain shielding can thus be expected and
may present itself as a long- term problem. The incidence, extent and consequences
may be the deciding factors in the future developments. Lack or loss of proximal
stem support, and the consequent stem fracture, was the midterm problem.

As stem fracture has been largely eliminated by improved materials, design and
cementing technique the proximal strain shielding can be expected to present later,
past the 11 year follow-up. It was during the 11 year follow-up that the Charnley flat
back stems that failed, did so.

Fig. 20.17 Radiograph of
a collared femoral stem
with fracture

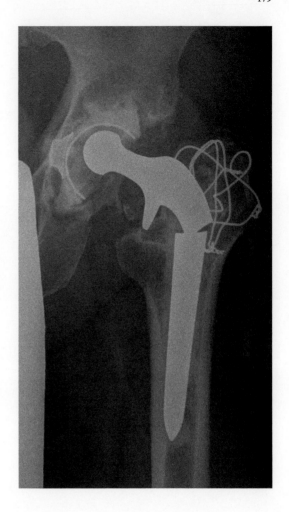

Reference

1. Wroblewski BM. Revision surgery in total hip arthroplasty. London: Springer; 1990.
   p. 136–7.

Chapter 21
Patterns of Failure of Stem Fixation

Use of radio-opaque cement and availability of good quality serial radiographs, showing all of the stem and cement, is essential in order to study the patterns of failure of stem fixation. The three basic patterns can be recognised: slip, tilt and pivot. Although obvious, when typical, an overlap between the types is common.

Slip

Stem Within the Cement Mantle

Limited taper slip of the stem within the cement mantle is the principle behind the design of the C-Stem and the surgical technique of stem fixation. The slip can be recognised, radiologically, by the separation of the stem from the cement proximally on the lateral aspect (Fig. 21.1).

If the stem was supported distally by cement then fracture of the cement at the tip of the stem will be seen [1] (Fig. 21.2).

These changes may be observed early, usually within the first post-operative year. They may be innocuous. The problem, however, is the real possibility of fragmentation of the cement in the proximal medial region. Regular monitoring is essential. Such changes may herald endosteal cavitation, stem loosening or fracture.

Stem Between the Layers of Cement

Invariably a result of inadequate exposure, preparation of the femur, cementing technique and stem insertion. Limited exposure and entry through the neck of the femur directing the stem posteriorly. Common presentation of early technical failure more obvious on lateral radiographs (Fig. 21.3). Beware of periprosthetic fracture of the femur!

© Springer International Publishing Switzerland 2016

B.M. Wroblewski et al., *Charnley Low-Frictional Torque Arthroplasty of the Hip: Practice and Results*, DOI 10.1007/978-3-319-21320-0_21

Fig. 21.1 Radiograph
showing a slip of the
femoral stem within
cement mantle. Separation
of stem from cement
denotes stem slip or/and
stem tilt into varus

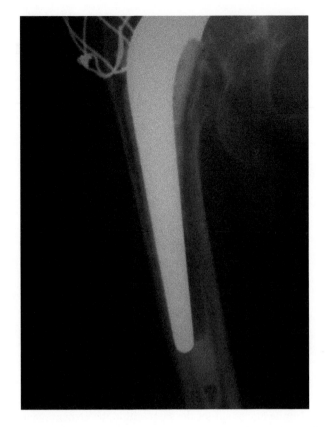

Stem-Cement Complex

The failure occurs at the bone-cement interface and infection should be excluded. If purely mechanical it is slowly progressive and invariably in conjunction with a rough surface finish of the stem.

Tilt

Tilt of the Stem

This is almost invariably the result of an inadequate stem fixation. It is basically a tilt of the stem into varus and retroversion (Fig. 21.1)

Fig. 21.2 Radiograph
showing fracture cement at
the tip of the femoral stem,
separation of stem from
cement and endosteal
cavitation medially

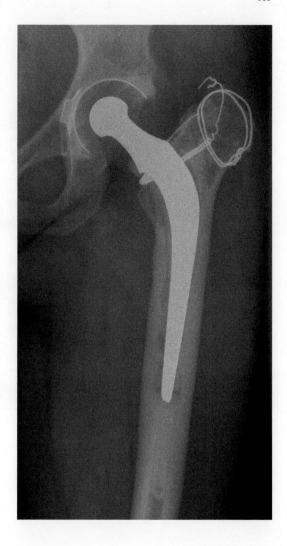

Tilt of the Stem-Cement Complex

En masse, it is almost invariably due to deep infection. Clinical observation suggests that, even in the presence of deep infection, the better the cementing technique the later this mechanism of failure presents itself (Fig. 21.4).

Fig. 21.3 Radiograph
showing slip of the femoral
stem between cement
layers. This is a result of
inadequate exposure and
preparation of the
medullary canal

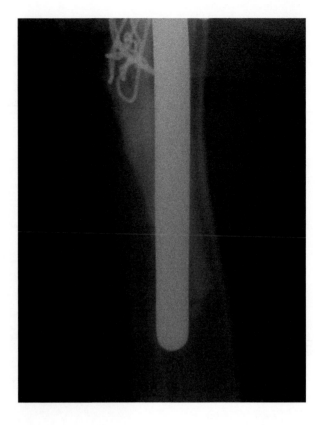

Pivot

Two radiographic patterns can be distinguished: stem within the distal cement and
stem tip on a distal cement column.

Stem Within Distal Cement

Is the result of stem slip/subsidence within the cement with destruction of the proximal cement mantle. Progressive proximal endosteal cavitation is the pattern and
may lead to periprosthetic fracture of the femur (Fig. 21.2).

Stem Tip on Distal Cement

With the stem supported distally on a column of cement there may be, initially
gradual, but eventually rapidly progressive, endosteal cavitation starting proximally.
It is with these changes that periprosthetic fractures occur (Fig. 21.5).

Fig. 21.4 Radiograph
showing tilting of femoral
stem cement complex.
Infection suspected

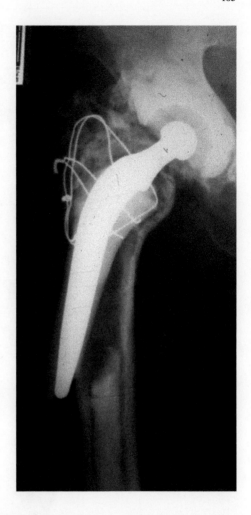

It may be of practical interest to point out a detail concerning setting of cement
during surgery. Cement does not set uniformly; it sets from the bone towards the
implant, from distal to proximal. If after insertion of the stem the stem is moved, it
will open the cement mantle – proximally. This would result in the stem being supported distally but free to move within the cement mantle proximally.

Recognition of the patterns of failure is of interest in planning follow-up and
operative interventions. The skill lies in their prevention by the selection of correct
stem designs and correct surgical technique with the use of cement

Fig. 21.5 Radiograph of
femoral stem pivoting and
supported by a distal
cement column. Endosteal
cavitation – periprosthetic
fracture is the likely
outcome. The cup is well
fixed with minimal wear

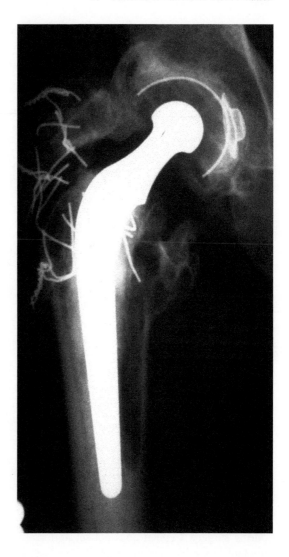

Reference

1. Weber FA, Charnley J. A radiological study of fractures of acrylic cement in relation to the
   stem of the femoral head prosthesis. J Bone Joint Surg (Br). 1975;57-B:297–301.

Chapter 22
Fracture of the Stem

In this clinic, within a period of 2 years and after more than 10 years experience with total hip replacement, the fatigue fracture of the metal of the stem of the femoral prosthesis revealed itself as a definite complication of the operation, and not even an incident of such extreme rarity as hardly to offer a serious problem. (1975)

Charnley's statement summarizes the effect this complication presented. This, in a way, is not unexpected. The process leading up to the fracture of the stem, or in fact any process especially one spanning a number of years, does not have the same effect as an event. This distinction, between a process and an event, is the essential aspect of the study of long-term results in total hip arthroplasty. In order to chart a process, regular review and recording of information is essential. In joint replacement surgery this demands, not only regular follow-up, but also a collection of detailed and meaningful data which can be used, not merely for research purposes, but more importantly for improvements to be made. Recording the end point, fracture of the stem or a single indication for a revision may be interesting but it fails to provide the vital information concerning the processes leading up to the event – the revision.

Fracture of the original "flat back" Charnley stem in stainless steel, EN58J, was the event that stimulated further research and development of new materials, designs and surgical technique. It may be of interest to recall Charnley's comment once the initial surprise has passed: *"And I thought there was nothing else to do."* So what was the information gathered as the result of a clinical study of the first 17 fractured stems?

Clinical Findings [1]

All, except two fractures occurred in males. The mean age at primary LFA was 60 years (26–82). Their mean weight was 86 kg (57–109). All patients *"...had recovered functional capacity equal to that of normal people of the same age."*

© Springer International Publishing Switzerland 2016

B.M. Wroblewski et al., *Charnley Low-Frictional Torque Arthroplasty of the Hip: Practice and Results*, DOI 10.1007/978-3-319-21320-0_22

In five cases there was a history of trauma "*... with the onset of definitive symptoms but almost certainly this ... indicated a creeping crack becoming complete.*"

Radiological Findings

– Position of the stem within the medullary canal was: varus in 9, neutral in 6 and valgus in 2.
– Imperfect support (of the stem) by cement presenting as fracture of the cement at the tip of the stem, or separation of the proximal–lateral border of the stem, was observed in seven cases.
– The level of the fracture of the stem was between 7 and 10.5 cm from the tip: the segment as risk, measuring 3.5 cm.
– Erosion at the level of the medial aspect of the femoral neck, causing defective support of the prosthesis by the cement was considered to be – probably – a universal finding and the cause of fracture of the stem.
– At surgery – fragmentation of the cement at the medial femoral neck area was always visible. Whether this was the cause or the effect of the fracture could not be established at surgery. But, taking this finding in conjunction with detailed history, fragmentation of cement must have occurred before stem fracture.

(For a stem to subside within the cement mantle, as with fracture of the cement at the tip of the stem, and to separation from the cement mantle – proximally laterally – proximal medial femoral cement may, at times, fragment. If this cement remains intact and continues to support the stem, the stem will migrate distally with the tip approaching the medial femoral cortex and, therefore, less likely to have moved medially proximally).

> *The mechanical situation which would favour fatigue fracture of a prosthesis is defective support by the layer of cement which is interposed between the bone of the calcar and the concave upper part of the stem ...when this is combined with the firm bonding of the lower part of the stem...*

These findings also indicate that distal stem fixation, within the cement, can be near perfect.

Summary

The problem leading to stem fracture was: lack or loss of proximal stem support in the presence of good distal stem fixation. The dimensions of the standard "flat back" stem in EN58J stainless steel were considered inadequate for patients over 77 kg weight [1].

Further Studies of Fracture of the Stem [2]

The review of records of 120 cases of fractures Charnley "flat back" stems has revealed the following information:

- The period "at risk" for stem fracture was 11 years from the time of the operation and 97.5 % fractured during that time. Early fractures occurring during the second to fourth year were usually in revisions for a previous stem fracture. If corrosion is a <u>progressive destruction</u> of metal by body fluids, and stainless steel has the fatigue limit characteristic, then the suggestion is that the body environment is non-corrosive. If this interpretation is correct then use of "corrosion resistant" materials does not seem to be justified.
- There was a linear relationship between patients' weight and the time of the fracture.
- Radiographic evidence of the failure of full stem fixation was found in 77.2 % of cases where serial radiographs were available.
- Loss of proximal stem support, as judged the height of the neck of the femur, was present in 73.3 %.
- In patients of comparable weight, stems in valgus position fractured earlier than those in varus position.
- Patients of comparable weight, and referred from other units, fractured the stem significantly earlier.
- It was considered that the patients' weight limit for this particular prosthesis should be 66 kg (145 lbs) which was much lower than the 77 kg suggested by Charnley [1].

The Mechanism of Stem Fracture

"Examination of 70 fractured Charnley flat back femoral prostheses, suggested that the causative mechanism was a torsional loading of the proximal portion on the distal part of the stem" [3]

Components collected at revision surgery have always served as "flight recorders"; an invaluable research material. Together with clinical data and good quality radiographs available from regular follow-up, they served as excellent material for modifications and improvements in the design, materials and surgical technique.

Results of the Study

Examination of 70 fractured stems revealed the following information:-

Obliquity of the Fracture (Figs. 22.1 and 22.2)

Viewed from the lateral aspect the fracture line was always at an angle to the long axis of the stem. From the direction of the obliquity it was possible to determine the side from which the specimen was retrieved; the obliquity was always upwards away from the operated side. The degree of the slope varied from 2 to 20° with an average of 9.9°. The degree of the slope of the fracture was considered to reflect and be proportional to, the length of the stride, assuming of course that the stem remained positioned in the coronal plane.

Bending of the Proximal Fragment (Fig. 22.3)

The proximal fragment was rotated downwards and backwards in relation to the distal fragment.

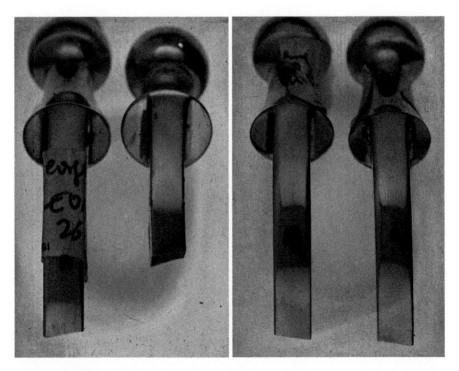

Figs. 22.1 and 22.2 Obliquity of fracture line, viewed from the lateral aspect, identifies the site – *left* or *right* (Reproduced from Wroblewski [9])

Fig. 22.3 Bending torsion
of the proximal fragment
in relation to the fixed
distal part of the stem.
(Left hip) (Reproduced
from Wroblewski [9])

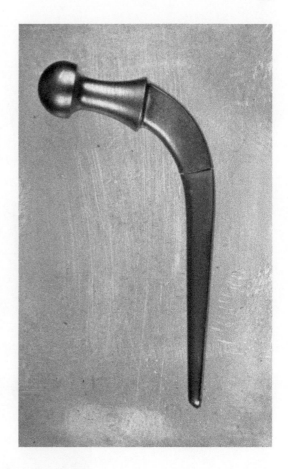

Fracture Wave (Tide Marks) (Fig. 22.4)

If the revision was carried out soon after the fracture had occurred, it was possible to identify the origin of the fracture. This was always adjacent to the relatively square antero-lateral corner of the stem and extended proximally, posteriorly, and medially. The spacing of the waves was thought to correspond to individual loads which exceeded a certain level and resulted in the propagation of the fracture wave. If this reasoning is correct then counting the individual waves would suggest the number of loads to the final failure, while their spacing the magnitude of each load.

Fracture Lip (Fig. 22.5)

This was the remnant of the metal, invariably on the medial margin of the stem, the last portion of the stem that failed suddenly, "… *indicated creeping crack becoming complete* …"

Fig. 22.4 Fatigue fracture
wave – the origin of the
fracture is at the antero-
lateral margin of the stem
(Reproduced from
Wroblewski [9])

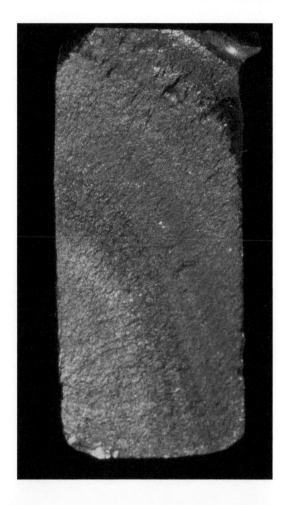

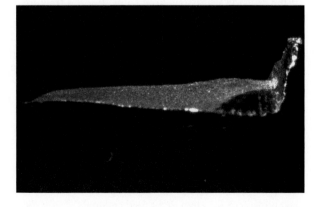

Fig. 22.5 Fracture
lip – denotes sudden
failure of the femoral stem
as it is unable to sustain the
load (Reproduced from
Wroblewski [9])

Level of the Fracture (Figs. 22.6 and 22.7)

The upper limit of the level of the fracture corresponded with the portion of the stem where the curve of the stem had its beginning – all fractures occurred below that level. The segment of the 45 mm offset stem, at risk of a fracture, was about 4 cm long: 5.5–9.5 cm from the tip of the stem. For the 37.5 mm offset stem the segment it was 2 cm long: 9–11 cm from the tip for the stem. Straighter stems fractured more proximally with a shorter segment at risk for fracture.

Conclusion

"Fracture of the stem is but a dramatic presentation of the end result of loosening of the proximal part of the stem in the presence of good distal fixation [1]

The information gathered indicated that the pattern of stem fracture reflected the function of the hip whereby the load is from the antero-superior direction; the hip is loaded in flexion and the load is out of plane of the neck of the femur. The fracture starts at the antero-lateral margin and extends proximally, posteriorly and medially. This could explain the mechanism in other hip pathologies.

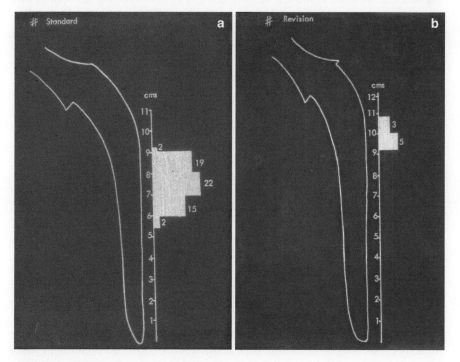

Figs. 22.6 and 22.7 Level of stem fracture depending on offset. (**a**) 45 mm offset. (**b**) 37.5 mm offset (Reproduced from Wroblewski [9])

- Perthes disease of the hip with the antero-superior quadrant of the femoral head as a site of the early disease process.
- Slipped upper femoral epiphysis, with the slip usually taking place gradually, at times with a sudden progression, the epiphysis migrating postero-medially.
- Avascular necrosis of the femoral head, like Perthe's disease, located initially, in the antero-superior quadrant: suggesting "load located" lesions.
- Fracture of the neck of the femur, with the postero-medial comminution clearly confirms the pattern of the load on the hip joint as a functional and not a static pathology.
- Some cases of osteoarthritis where the early sign is the narrowing of joint space, antero-superiorly – seen on a lateral radiograph.

Fracture of the Stem: Further Information

The classical pattern of stem fracture, as previously documented [3] has offered invaluable information concerning design, materials and the surgical technique of stem fixation. It also focused the attention on the mechanical aspects of some hip pathologies. With time and improvements the incidence declined rapidly; the interest in the complication ceased. In its place came, first the stem loosening, then because of the lack of regular follow-up and early revision, periprosthetic fractures of the femur.

It may not be out of place to bring to notice three further modes of stem fracture: hinging, impingement and valgus. These patterns bring further information concerning hip function in general and total hip arthroplasty in particular.

Hinging out of a total of 220 revisions for stem fracture, 15 (6.8 %) had a further stem fracture [4]. All but one were in males, all were over 85 kg (187 lbs). The unusual finding at revision was the mass of cement still adherent to the proximal fragment. The explanation is in the details of the revision. After removal of the distal fragment and the cement, the proximal femur was not prepared adequately for cement injection. The lesser trochanter was not excavated to offer good quality cancellous bone offering support for the stem postero-medially. The distal cement was not cleared sufficiently; the end to end junction between the old and the new cement became a "fault line" failing early.

The proximal part of the stem, supported on the new cement now hinged on the junction with the old cement, literally tearing the stem apart (Figs. 22.8, 22.9, 22.10, and 22.12).

The mechanism was confirmed experimentally. It was also found, again, in clinical practice with collared stems: this time the collar functioning as a hinge (Fig. 20.17).

Impingement of the neck of the stem on the rim of the cup may appear to be an unlikely cause of stem fracture but such a case was documented with the Ring metal on metal prosthesis [4]. Because of component orientation, cup retroversion, the neck of the stem impinged on the anterior rim of the cup. The proximal part of the

Fig. 22.8 Radiograph showing a femoral stem fracture

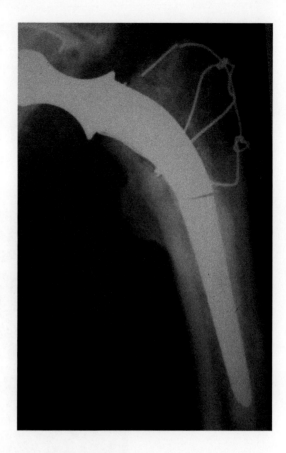

stem now becomes "fixed" while the shaft of the femur continues in its forward motion striking the stem from behind. The obliquity of the fracture would be the reverse from the common pattern reported [4]. Neck erosion in metal on metal hip resurfacing may be due to impingement of the neck of the femur on the rim of the cup. The explanation could be very simple. The natural acetabulum is asymmetric both in structure and function: it allows freedom of movement without impingement. A symmetrical cup in resurfacing does no cater for that – cup orientation now depends on the surgeon's skill. Impingement, neck erosion and fracture could be the result.

"Valgus" stem fracture is a new entity and yet offers an insight into some cases of femoral neck fracture. Findings of incomplete stem fracture at revision has not been common [4], while a fracture originating on the medial aspect of the stem has not been reported before. An incidental finding at revision – for cup wear and loosening – shows clearly the valgus position of the proximal fragment (Fig. 22.11). Is the mechanism similar to that of an impacted, valgus fracture of the neck of the femur; completion of the fracture and a fall rather than a fall causing the fracture? This question has been posed before. Reeves [5] asked this question: "What comes first, the fracture of the fall?" He concluded that "…there was a group of elderly

Fig. 22.9 The mechanism
was in clinical practice
with collared stems: this
time the collar functioning
as a hinge

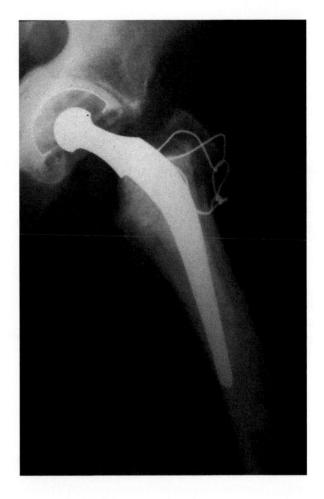

patients … in whom fracture of the femoral neck occurred under the loads imparted during quiet walking."

If a total hip arthroplasty restores normal function there is no reason to doubt why the consequences should be any other but similar in both the natural and the artificial. Clearly a scope for further research.

Fracture of the Stem: Temperatures Generated and the Possible Implications

Fracture of the stem in primary total hip arthroplasty (THA) is now largely of historical interest. The mechanism: bending-torsion was documented [6] its role in other "load located" lesion highlighted [7], and the clinical aspects of 120 cases published [8].

Fig. 22.10 The mechanism was in clinical practice with collared stems: this time the collar functioning as a hinge. (See Fig. 20.17 for Radiograph of fractured collared stem)

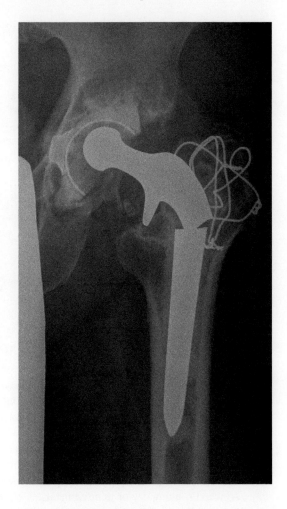

In a collection of 70 fractured stems which formed the basis of the study of the mechanism of fracture [6], there was 56 where the fracture wave was clearly visible. The origin of the fracture was at or near the antero-lateral corner of the stem. In two stems, where the fracture wave was preserved, colour change: the "rainbow" effect was observed. Both stems were of the Charnley "flat back" design with a polished surface finish.

The colour spectrum showed a range from yellow-brown to purple-red with a suggestion of transition to grey (Fig. 22.13). Colour changes associated with various temperatures are given for comparison (Fig. 22.14) and would suggest that temperatures of 250–280 °C and maybe even higher, are generated during the process of fatigue fracture of the stem.

It should not come as a surprise that failure of a stem by fatigue, like any other metal, should generate high temperatures locally. Could it be that closely packed fracture waves indicate high frequency of loading, each load exceeding the fatigue

Fig. 22.11 "Valgus" stem
fracture. Incomplete
fracture originating on the
medial surface. Proximal
fragment shows valgus
shift

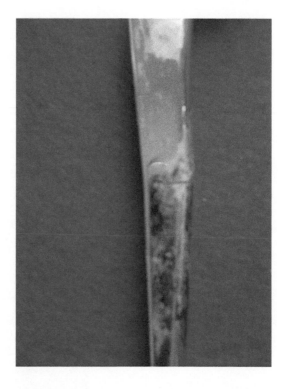

strength of the intact portion of the stem, without the time delay to dissipate the
temperature? Possibility of temperature generation at the level of the artificial articulation, during activity, has not received detailed attention. Our observation suggests that a rise of over 250 °C appear to have been reached locally. If our findings
are confirmed then the implications must be considered. What would the consequences be if such high temperatures were generated at the level of the articulation,
more so when running dry or in circumstances with reduced possibility of heat dis-
sipation as with ceramics with their insulating properties?

Study of "high activity" levels in patients after total hip arthroplasty may take us
beyond the assessment by the accepted clinical parameters and into the sphere of
detailed mechanics of the new articulation.

Fig. 22.12 Radiograph showing a stem fracture with the stem in valgus position, cement mass with proximal fragment medially

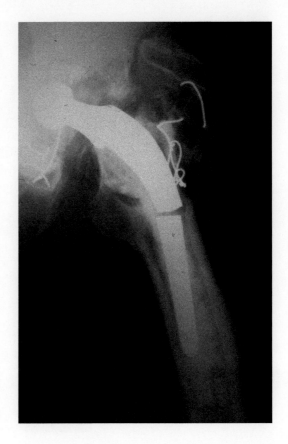

Fig. 22.13 Fracture
surface showing colour
bands (Reproduced from
Wroblewski [9])

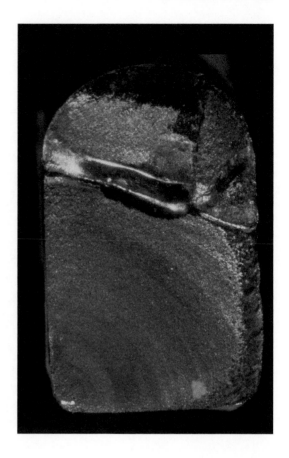

Centigrade

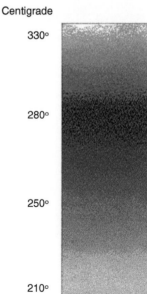

Fig. 22.14 Colour bands with associated temperatures

References

1. Charnley J. Fracture of femoral prostheses in total hip replacement. A clinical study. Clin Orthop Relat Res. 1975;111:105–20.
2. Wroblewski BM. Fracture of the stem in total hip replacement. A clinical review of 120 cases. Acta Orthop Scand. 1982;53:279–84.
3. Wroblewski BM. The mechanism of fracture of the femoral prosthesis in total hip replacement. Int Orthop (SICOT). 1979;3:137–9.
4. Wroblewski BM. Revision surgery in total hip arthroplasty. London: Springer; 1990. p. 125–38.
5. Reeves B. What comes first, the fracture or the fall? A study of subcapital fractures. J Bone Joint Surg (Br). 1977;59-B:375.
6. Wroblewski BM. The mechanism of fracture of the femoral prosthesis in total hip replacement. SICOT Int Orthop. 1979;3:137–9.
7. Wroblewski BM. Transverse load on the hip joint: a subject for further research. Eng Med. 1980;9(3):163–4.
8. Wroblewski BM. Fractured stem in total hip replacement. A clinical review of 120 cases. Acta Orthop. 1982;53:279–84.
9. Wroblewski BM. Revision surgery in total hip arthroplasty. London: Springer; 1990. p. 131–5.

Chapter 23
Intramedullary Cancellous Bone Block

The concept of closing off the medullary canal, distal to the planned stem position, was considered to be a relatively simple method of achieving containment of the cement and its pressurization using the two thumb method. Four possible materials could be used: metal, cement, UHMWPE or bone: all were considered, the first three very briefly.

Metal either solid or a mesh type restrictor, would have had the problem of its extraction at revision. In contact with the stem would invite fretting.

Cement restrictors would demand a range of sizes, instrumentation inventory and all the problems associated with it. Flexible cement restrictors were experimented with. Composition of the cement was altered to give a relatively flexible shuttlecock-type restrictor. The idea was reasonable but it's execution met with difficulties. The formulation of a suitable cement mix proved difficult; the end product's properties were temperature dependent. It worked well when warm but became brittle when cold. At surgery it showed its visco-elastic properties rather dramatically: a slight tap on the introducer would shatter the restrictor.

UHMWPE was the obvious choice, but not without possible long-term problems. A solid restrictor would have to carry with it instrumentation for measuring the medullary canal before the appropriate size could be chosen and placed at a correct level. The chosen size would only fit at a certain level – which may not be under the surgeon's control. A shuttlecock-type design was obvious, its manufacture less so. Insertion down the medullary canal would invite abrasion of UHMWPE against cancellous bone and shedding of plastic particles. (This fact became obvious when there were opportunities to revise some loose stems when this design had been used: "petals" of the plastic could be found anywhere from the level of the greater trochanter down to the distal cement). Removal of such a device was not easy: designed to close on insertion it would tend to open on extraction! If failures were to present in the future, and if tissue reaction to UHMWPE wear particles did prove to be the cause of the problem, then clearly UHMWPE was best avoided; cavitation at the tip of the stem would demand by-passing the defect with a longer stem.

© Springer International Publishing Switzerland 2016
B.M. Wroblewski et al., *Charnley Low-Frictional Torque Arthroplasty of the Hip: Practice and Results*, DOI 10.1007/978-3-319-21320-0_23

Design, Instrumentation and Clinical Application

A trephine to take the bone block either from the sectioned neck or the femoral head, the neck of the femur at the neck-trochanteric junction – or from all three areas if needs be. The trephine must allow easy ejection of the bone block (Fig. 23.1).

A set of tampers which could be used, first to measure the diameter of the medullary canal at certain depths, and then to allow distal impaction of the bone block.

Clinical experience dictated that a 15 mm diameter bone block would serve most cases, except the extremely narrow canals or the exceptionally wide ones. For the extremely narrow ones, a paediatric bone block set was designed – 10 mm diameter. For the exceptionally wide ones, extra bone was used from a disc of bone taken from the femoral neck. Clinical experience, again, dictated that tampers 8, 10, 12 and 14 mm diameter would serve the purpose (Fig. 23.2).

Clinical application of the method gave immediate indication of the pressures that could be generated when introducing the stem. The post-operative radiographs invited comments concerning neatly cut off cement down the medullary canal.

At this stage of evolution the cement was packed down the medullary canal using the two-thumb method. If the first lot of cement was pushed rather far the next wave would trap air which could be heard to pop when the stem was introduced. No doubt air was also trapped within the medullary canal – between the bone block and the first introduction of cement. The medullary canal had to be vented.

A vent with an obturator was designed (Fig. 23.3). The vent was inserted to the level of the bone block and the obturator was withdrawn, the cement was thumbed down the medullary canal. When fully packed the vent was occluded with the thumb

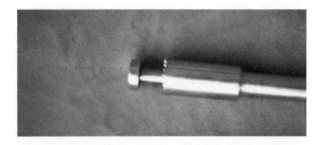

Fig. 23.1 A trephine to take the bone block either from the sectioned neck or the femoral head. The instrument allows easy ejection of the bone block

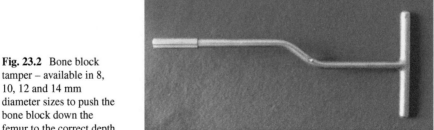

Fig. 23.2 Bone block tamper – available in 8, 10, 12 and 14 mm diameter sizes to push the bone block down the femur to the correct depth

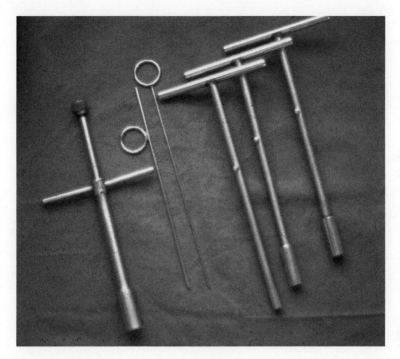

Fig. 23.3 Intramedullary bone block. Set of instruments

to prevent sucking back of its contents, and withdrawn. The cement was pressurised again before stem insertion. The alternative is to deliver cement from distal to proximal using a cement gun.

The idea of the intramedullary cancellous bone block being introduced into clinical practice had other aims for future developments – and not just improving cement injection. The plan was to address the whole concept of the function of the cemented stem. The stimulus was fracture of the stem which was studied in some detail. The problem was lack or loss of proximal stem support in the presence of distal stem fixation.

Intramedullary bone block, when placed at the correct level, allowed the tip of the stem to penetrate into it thus avoiding distal stem support allowing limited stem slip within the cement mantle. The design and the technique were deliberate to achieve this aim. "… it may be possible to dispense altogether with cement distal to the prosthesis" [1]. (Note the early plans in the development of the C-Stem.)

Reference

1. Wroblewski BM, van der Rijt AJ. Intramedullary cancellous bone block to improve femoral stem fixation in Charnley low friction arthroplasty. J Bone Joint Surg (Br). 1984;66-B:639–44.

Chapter 24
Loosening of the Stem

From the brief description of the role of the femoral component in general, and its intramedullary portion in particular, it is clear that loosening of the stem may be anticipated. It is the detailed study of failures that is an essential aspect of continuing evolution of the Charnley concept.

Inadequate Fixation

The aim of total hip arthroplasty is not only pain relief but also restoration of patient's activity level. Walking is the highest load to which the hip joint is subjected, other than occasionally. It must, therefore, follow that in some situations fixation of the stem may prove inadequate and loosening may result. Single episode resulting in failure is certainly dramatic but fortunately relatively rare. Accumulation of damage over a period of time is insidious and may, and often does, pass unnoticed. Some of the clinical situations can be modelled experimentally. The RSA technique is most valuable in the measurement of the very minor changes of position of an implant within the skeleton. (The principle of the method known for millennia as "celestial parallax").

The method aims to measure the earliest changes of the position of the implant within the skeleton. It is, therefore, reasonable to suggest that it should be used first to establish the validity of the method as applied to the concept under investigation. Next it should be used experimentally, to test the surgeon's ability to consistently achieve the result. Only when this has been achieved should it be applied clinically. To miss the first two stages is not only to miss the earliest of changes that can and do occur under clinical conditions, but also to assume that the surgeon's skill is not at fault.

The RSA technique should not be used to vindicate surgical technique and condemn the implant.

© Springer International Publishing Switzerland 2016 207
B.M. Wroblewski et al., *Charnley Low-Frictional Torque Arthroplasty of the Hip: Practice and Results*, DOI 10.1007/978-3-319-21320-0_24

Fatigue and wear testing of components are routine though the details of methods may vary. What cannot be reproduced adequately, experimentally, is the changing quality of the skeleton and the changes that the implant may impose on the skeleton. It is for those reasons that regular follow-up with good quality radiographs, and continuity of observer method, are essential. Combined with detailed documentation of surgical technique they will allow identification of both advantageous and problematic features of design, material and surgical technique.

Excluding infection, early mechanical loosening, within the first year or 2, could be due to the inadequate component fixation. It may not be indicative of a failure of the method but certainly of that particular procedure, for that particular patient by that particular surgeon. Adequate training in the technique and regular performance of the procedure and **regular review of the results are essential**.

Excessive Loading

If we assume that surgical technique can be standardised and uniformly applied at every operation, then we have to accept that the same principle is unlikely to apply to the quality of bone stock available or the patient's activity level. It is the loading pattern that would eventually identify the patients at risk. It could be surmised that heavy males with a unilateral hip problem and no other activity restricting factors (Charnley category A cases) will be at greater risk for stem loosening.

Strain Shielding

Introducing a load bearing stem will alter the pattern of load transfer: proximal strain shielding and distal strain concentration. Proximally this presents as loss of cortical definition especially of the medial femoral neck, loss of height (Fig. 24.1) and breadth of cortex, distal cortical hypertrophy (Fig. 24.2), is the evidence of strain concentration.

Progressive loss of proximal stem support would result in increasing amplitude of stem deflection under load. Circulating bursal fluid and its contents, subject to pressure and volume changes, would lead to mechanical erosion at the bone-implant interface on the femoral side (Fig. 24.1) and on the acetabular side (Fig. 24.3). The end result may be stem loosening or fracture of the stem (Fig. 24.2). If revision is delayed then periprosthetic fracture of the femur will be the consequence.

Loosening of the Stem: Radiographic Appearances

When assessing radiographic appearances of the cemented components it is essential that the cement is made radiopaque. [1] Initially, in a handful of cases, this was not so. The information that could be obtained was limited. Charnley introduced

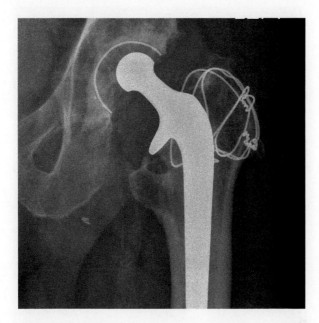

Fig. 24.1 Radiograph showing collared femoral stem with loss of cortical height of medial femoral neck

barium sulphate powder for the purpose of rendering the cement radio-opaque. The powder was contained in 2 g cachets together with tablets of formaldehyde – as a method of sterilisation. Barium sulphate was added to the polymer powder, one packet for the acetabulum and two for the femur, before mixing it with the monomer. (The quantity of barium sulphate added was in accord with the radio-density of bone and thus produced a more comparable appearance. The quality of dispersal of the powder was also taken as a reflection of the mixing skill of the theatre staff). Some of the appearances may already be anticipated from the description of mechanism of failure of stem fracture.

Pacheco at al. [2] reviewed radiographs of 72 revisions for aseptic stem loosening describing the radiographic appearances at 1 year and comparing them with those in a group of 116 clinically successful LFAs. The follow-up was 7.7 years (1–17) to revision and 15–21 years in the clinically successful cases.

The results are shown in Table 24.1: together with statistical significance.

Three aspects of any such a study must be appreciated. First that each of the radiographic appearances does not usually occur in isolation but are a reflection of more complex inter-related changes taking place in space. Second, a radiographic appearance may be looked on as an event presenting at a certain stage of a process. Thus, demarcation or condensation of bone at the tip of the stem, or endosteal cavitation, take time to develop. The timing of the findings will depend on the frequency of the radiographs being taken. Furthermore, the presentation on a radiograph will be masked by the radio-density of the femoral cortex. It is only when the increase –

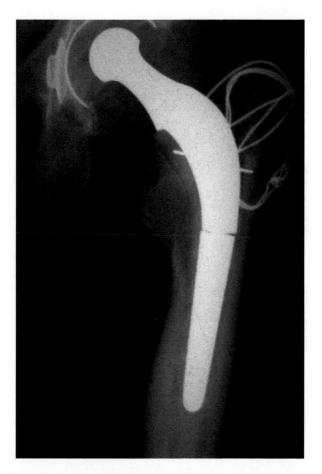

Fig. 24.2 Radiograph showing proximal strain shielding and distal strain concentration. Proximally this presents as loss of cortical definition and stem fracture

condensation – or decrease – e.g. endosteal cavitation – reaches the extent which can be "seen through the femoral cortex" that it is recorded as "being present". The condensation of bone, frequently referred to as pedestal, must reach the density of two layers of femoral cortex – or even exceed it – before it is observed on radiographs. The same is true of endosteal cavitation, a certain proportion of cortical bone mass must be lost, and preferably over a localised area and with a well defined margin, for endosteal cavitation to be recorded as being present.

The third aspect is related to follow-up. A 1 year follow-up may give some indication of the future outcome, and may even be used as a guide in planning follow-up; practical experience dictates otherwise. Regular follow-up every 1–2 years up to 6 years is essential; it becomes interesting at 10 years. Five year intervals advocated by some are not based on evidence.

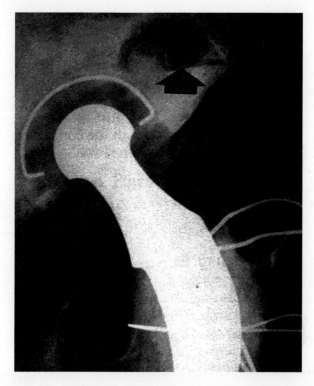

Fig. 24.3 Circulating bursal fluid and its contents, subject to pressure and volume changes, would lead to mechanical erosion at the bone-implant interface

Table 24.1 Radiographic appearances at 1 year of 72 cases revised for stem loosening compared with those of 116 clinically successful cases followed up for 15–21 years

Radiographic appearance at 1 year	72 revisions for stem loosening		116 successful cases		Statistical significance
	Number	%	Number	%	
Unchanged	12	16.7	70	60.3	p<0.002
Separation of stem from cement	19	26.4	31	26.7	
Demarcation at tip	43	59.7	21	18.1	p<0.001
Fracture tip of cement	12	16.7	4	3.4	p<0.001
Endosteal cavitation	1	1.4	0	0	
Stem position					
Varus	7	9.7	16	13.8	
Valgus	42	58.3	19	16.4	p<0.001
Neutral	23	31.9	81	69.8	p<0.002
Previous surgery	22	30.6	5	4.3	P<0.001

Stem Loosening: Clinical

Although clinical results do not reflect the mechanical state of the arthroplasty an attempt is made here to consider the likely mechanical changes resulting in a possible clinical problems.

The femur is viewed as a tubular closed system a "constant volume capacitor". Any condition tending to change the volume will have an effect of changing the intramedullary pressure. Experience dictates that an increase in the pressure will produce pain – a common feature in clinical practice and not just in orthopaedics. If a loose stem, with or without cement, creates a one way non-return valve system, it could be expected to become symptomatic when under load.

Conversely, a loose stem or one without fixation, may remain asymptomatic because the closed system has not been created. Erosion of the cortex by a tilting stem may be symptomatic, but if it is very gradual, it may remain unrecognised.

Failure of stem fixation, in the long term may be radiological, hence the need for regular radiographic checks is essential. It is the awareness of the problem and not the clinical results that will guide the surgeon as to the timing of the intervention by revision surgery. To delay revision and to await symptoms is to await periprosthetic fractures.

References

1. Weber FA, Charnley J. A radiological study of fractures of acrylic cement in relation to the stem of a femoral head prosthesis. J Bone Joint Surg (Br). 1975;57-B:297–301.
2. Pacheco V, Shelley P, Wroblewski BM. Mechanical loosening of the stem in Charnley arthroplasties. Identification of the "At Risk" factors. J Bone Joint Surg (Br). 1998;70-B:596–9.

Chapter 25
Position of the Stem Within the Medullary Canal

Position of the stem within the medullary canal in cemented total hip arthroplasties (THA) has been under scrutiny for some time. Initially this was in the context of stem fracture [1] then in relation to the predictability of the long-term outcome of stem fixation [2]. In both these publications only the antero-posterior (AP) radiographs were examined. More recently the attention has been focused on the high incidence of early failures [3] and suggestions made that endosteal cavitation and component loosening may be due to the direct effect of the ultra high molecular weight polyethylene (UHMWPE) wear particles gaining access to the bone cement interface through cement defects. As a result the trend in the design, instrumentation and the surgical technique has been to facilitate central placement of the stem within the medullary canal avoiding stem tip-cortex contact and aiming at a cement mantle of a predetermined thickness. To what extent does the position of the stem within the medullary canal in cemented THA play a part in the long-term outcome has not been established with certainty. Since a prospective study would not be possible, let alone acceptable, and a long-term follow-up would be necessary, [4] we have attempted to answer the question by examining both failed and successful cases retrospectively.

The review being retrospective it was not possible to comment on the cementing technique or the relevance of the cement mantle thickness as it was often disrupted by the process of loosening in the failed cases.

Successful result was defined as a patient who has had a cemented THA with a minimum follow-up of 8 years and considered the result to be clinically successful: the patient being free from the pre-operative hip pain, the hip having full or nearly full range of movement and the patient's activity level being normal or near normal for age, gender and the underlying hip pathology.

Failed result was defined as a patient who has had a revision for aseptic loosening of a cemented stem.

All the relevant information was extracted from the records and antero-posterior and lateral radiographs of the hip were examined. In the failed cases referred from other units, only the pre-revision AP and lateral radiographs were available.

© Springer International Publishing Switzerland 2016   213
B.M. Wroblewski et al., *Charnley Low-Frictional Torque Arthroplasty of the Hip: Practice and Results*, DOI 10.1007/978-3-319-21320-0_25

Definition of Stem Position

Antero-posterior Radiographs

<u>**Neutral position**</u> was defined when a line drawn through the centre of the shaft of the stem was in line with the centre of the medullary canal and an imaginary extension of the line drawn through the centre of the shaft of the stem would not encroach onto the femoral cortex as seen on the AP radiograph of the pelvis centred over the symphysis pubis (Fig. 25.1).

<u>**Valgus position**</u> was defined as the stem positioned laterally, within the medullary canal, in its proximal part with its distal end towards the medial femoral cortex, irrespective of whether or not the tip was touching or even encroaching into the medial femoral cortex (Fig. 25.2).

<u>**Varus position**</u> was when the stem was positioned towards the medial femoral neck proximally while its tip was directed towards the lateral femoral cortex, irrespective of whether or not it was touching or encroaching into the lateral femoral cortex (Fig. 25.3).

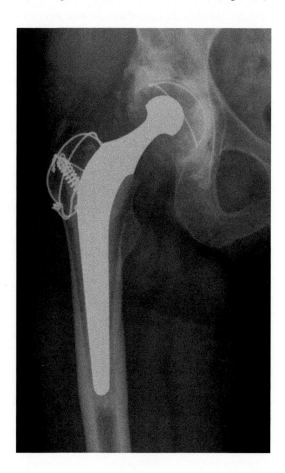

Fig. 25.1 Neutral stem position on an AP radiograph

Fig. 25.2 Valgus stem
position on an AP
radiograph

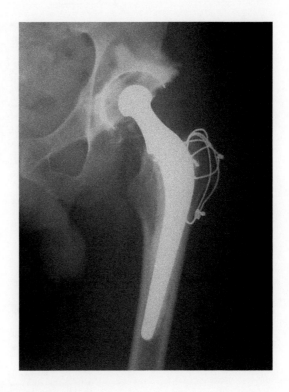

Lateral Radiographs

Neutral position as defined on the A.P. radiograph, (Fig. 25.4) but the radiograph was not centred over the symphysis pubis.

 Antero-posterior position was defined when the stem entered the medullary canal through or near the area of sectioned femoral neck and its tip was directed towards the posterior femoral cortex irrespective of whether it was touching or encroaching into the cortex (Fig. 25.5).

 Postero-anterior position was defined when the tip of the stem was directed towards the anterior cortex. irrespective of whether it was touching or encroaching into it (Fig. 25.6).

Results

Two hundred cemented THAs were reviewed: 100 clinically successful and 100 revised for aseptic stem loosening. Patients' details are shown in Table 25.1, the radiographic appearances in Tables 25.2, 25.3 and 25.4.

 Assessing the results we have used the Chi-square test.

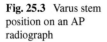

Fig. 25.3 Varus stem
position on an AP
radiograph

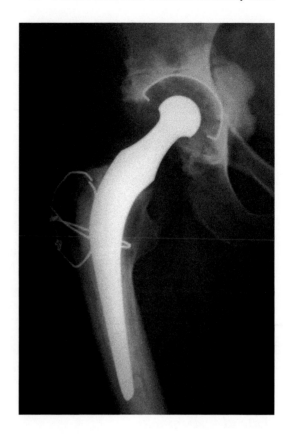

Discussion

If the position of the stem within the medullary canal in cemented THA be the only
indication of the long term success, then our findings suggest that a neutral orientation is desirable. In the successful group 77 were in neutral orientation on the
antero-posterior and 66 on the lateral radiograph; while 49 were in neutral orientation on both radiographs. In the failed group the corresponding numbers were 37
and 31 cases and only 9 were in a neutral orientation in both views (p < 0.0001).

Comparing stem alignment on both the antero-posterior and lateral radiographs
there is no statistical difference between the number of radiographs in each group:
211 in neutral and 189 in non-neutral alignment in the successful and revised cases
respectively. The number of radiographs with neutrally aligned stems in the successful group, 143, was significantly higher than the number of radiographs with
non-neutrally aligned stems, 57. The reverse was true of the revised group: there
were 68 radiographs with neutrally aligned stems but 132 radiographs with
non-neutrally aligned stems. The difference between the successful and the revised
group was statistically highly significant (p < 0.0001).

Fig. 25.4 View of lateral
radiograph with stem in
neutral position. Calcar
femorale not cleared

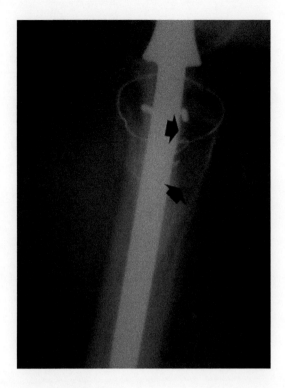

There was no evidence in the records to suggest that a particular position of the stem within the medullary canal was aimed for. The review is not meant to be a reflection of surgical technique of exposure, preparation of the medullary canal or cement injection, but merely of the stem position within the medullary canal.

The findings demand comment: the male to female ratio is reversed in the two groups. The most likely explanation could be that with a wider medullary canal in the male patient there is a greater chance of malposition of the stem unless the correct exposure and stem positioning is appreciated by the surgeon and a selection of stem sizes is made available. The patient's weight is probably also a contributory factor; the mean weight in the failed group was almost 10 kg higher.

To achieve central placement of the stem correct exposure of the medullary canal, not through the neck of the femur which encourages the stem to be directed posteriorly, but in the area of the piriformis fossa, is essential [5]. The preparation of the medullary canal, the role of the anatomical calcar [6] and the distal closure of the medullary canal [7] to improve stem fixation have been highlighted. It would be of benefit to individual surgeons to study both the antero-posterior and the lateral radiographs, post operatively, in order to assess the position of the stem as this may influence the long-term results.

The most likely explanation as to why the stem was placed in position other than neutral appears to be the access to the medullary canal; through the sectioned femo-

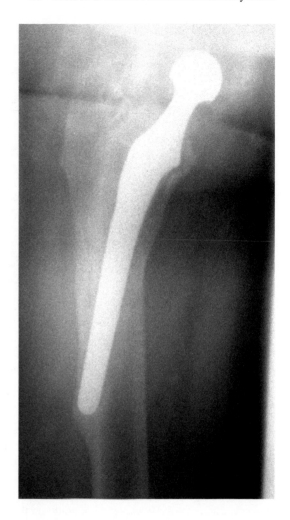

ral neck and not through the area of the piriform fossa. This was so in 90 out of 200 cases: 31 successful and 59 revised (p<0.001). This aspect has been pointed out before [5] and emphasised more recently [6].

Distal Stem Centralisers

The findings in this study question the role of distal centralisers: If a straight line is defined as the shortest distance between two points, can a "centraliser" attached to the tip of the stem, guide the stem into a central position when the point of entry is not in central alignment with the distal point? The answer must be in the negative.

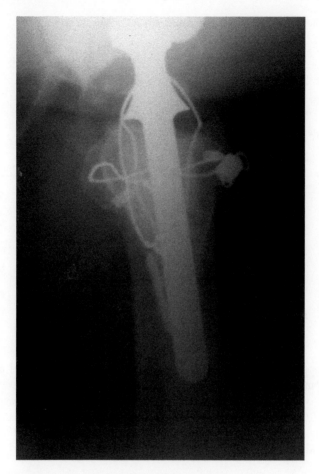

Fig. 25.6 View of lateral radiograph with stem positioned back to front

Table 25.1 Stem position – patient details

		Successful	Revised
Gender	Female	63	35
	Male	37	65
Age years/months	Mean	52/9	52/4
	Range	23–80/5	25/8–69/3
Weight/kg	Mean	66.3	75.7
	Range	47–102	50–110
Follow-up years/months	Mean	15/6	11/10
	Range	8/2–28/10	3/2–25/10

Table 25.2 Stem position and outcome (antero-posterior radiographs)

Stem position	Neutral		Valgus		Varus	
Outcome	Successful	Revised	Successful	Revised	Successful	Revised
Number of cases	77	37	17	43	6	20

Table 25.3 Stem position and outcome (lateral radiographs)

Stem position	Neutral		Valgus		Varus	
Outcome	Successful	Revised	Successful	Revised	Successful	Revised
Number of cases	66	31	31	59	3	10

Table 25.4 Stem alignment and outcome (AP and lateral radiographs)

Stem position	Neutral	Non-neutral
Number of radiographs	211	189
Successful, No (%)	143 (68)	57 (30)
Revised, No (%)	68 (32)	132 (70)

Correct exposure and preparation of the medullary canal is essential and merely placing a centraliser at the tip of the stem will not achieve this.

Position of the stem within the medullary canal is just but one aspect of the operation of total hip arthroplasty. Stem design and the technique of stem fixation using acrylic cement and the long-term results achieved with this method is a separate issue and discussed in other chapters.

References

1. Charnley J. Fracture of the femoral prosthesis in total hip replacement. A clinical study. Clin Orthop. 1975;111:105–20.
2. Pacheco V, Shelley P, Wroblewski BM. Mechanical loosening of the stem in Charnley arthroplasties. J Bone Joint Surg (Br). 1988;70-B:596–9.
3. Massoud SN, Hunter JB, Holdsworth BJ, Wallace WA, Juliusson R. Early femoral loosening in one design of cemented hip replacement. J Bone Joint Surg (Br). 1997;79-B:603–8.
4. Wroblewski BM, Fleming PA, Hall RM, Siney PD. Stem fixation in the Charnley low friction arthroplasty in young patients using an intramedullary bone block. J Bone Joint Surg (Br). 1998;80-B:273–8.
5. Wroblewski BM. Revision surgery in total hip arthroplasty. London: Springer; 1990. p. 17.
6. Wroblewski BM, Siney PD, Fleming PA, Bobak P. Calcar femoral: its role in cemented stem fixation in total hip arthroplasty. J Bone Joint Surg (Br). 2000;82-B:842–5.
7. Wroblewski BM, van der Rijt AJ. Intramedullary cancellous bone block to improve femoral stem fixation in Charnley low friction arthroplasty. J Bone Joint Surg (Br). 1984;66-B:639–44.

Chapter 26
C-Stem

The Concept, Design, Mechanical Testing, Surgical Technique and Results

It could be argued that we need "controlled subsidence" of the distal half of the stem to enable the cement in the upper end of the femur to maintain load-bearing contact with the cancellous bone. This might break the vicious circle, starting as elastic deformation of the upper end of the prosthesis too effectively supported below, and ending as granulomatous resorption of the medial femoral neck.

In 1968, 6 years after the introduction of the LFA into routine clinical practice, and after some 2500 operations have been carried out, stem fracture presented as a serious complication. The incidence peaked in the 8 year period 1974–1982. The attention focused on the stem design and the materials. The stem was made more bulky, angular corners were given a radius, and vaquasheening was used to work harden the surface and to ablate any irregularities that could act as possible stress risers. Proximal dorsal flange was added to improve cement injection. High nitrogen stainless steel was introduced, and the cold forming process gave a very strong material ORTRON (Chas. F. Thackray 1982) for stem manufacture. These changes, together with the technique of closing off the medullary canal with cancellous bone block [1] (October 1976) eliminated stem fracture. The incidence of aseptic stem loosening was also reduced with 99 % survivorship at 10 years in patients with a mean age of 41 years [2].

Regular reviews of radiographs of these clinically successful cases highlighted changes in the proximal femur indicating strain shielding. The process, no longer interrupted by stem fracture, now continued past the 11-year "at risk" period. It was totally asymptomatic.

It is the observation and interpretation of the radiographic changes of the proximal femur, first with stem fracture, then aseptic stem loosening and finally proximal strain shielding of the femur, were the reasons for the design of the C-Stem and the detailed attention to the cementing technique [3].

© Springer International Publishing Switzerland 2016   221
B.M. Wroblewski et al., *Charnley Low-Frictional Torque Arthroplasty of the Hip: Practice and Results*, DOI 10.1007/978-3-319-21320-0_26

The insertion of the intramedullary stem alters the pattern of load transfer to the femur; the consequence is the proximal strain shielding and distal strain concentration.

As a result of these changes the elasticity of the proximal femur increases and so does the amplitude of deflection of the stem – cement complex *"ending as granulamatous resorption of the medial femoral neck,"* bone erosion and cavitation – commonly referred to as osteolysis.

The Design

Incorporates the triple taper: antero-posterior, lateral to medial and proximal to distal – continuous throughout the intramedullary part of the stem. (Fig. 20.6) Broad, rounded lateral surface presents the bulk of metal for strength. The broad proximal portion resists torsion. Continuous tapers and polished surface allows engagement within the cement mantle when under load. Distal stem support is avoided by the tip of the stem entering the intramedullary bone-block which allows pressurisation of cement.

The surgical technique places the demand on the cementing technique from the exposure, to preparation of the medullary canal with particular attention to the calcar femorale.

Experimental Studies

A number of studies were carried out independently with DePuy International (Leeds U.K.) holding the information. The aspects examined subsidence, stress analysis, changes in the bone strain pattern and comparison with various stem designs available commercially.

Early Results

In the initial publication 500 primary operations were analysed at a mean follow-up of 3 years and 5 months (1–7 years). There were no revisions for stem loosening and no stem was considered to be at risk for loosening. In 20 % there was radiological evidence of improvement in the quality of the bone-cement interface [3].

Long-Term Results

Since the introduction of the C-Stem into routine clinical practice in November 1993 – 7429 have been implanted of which 6033 are primaries and 1396 revisions.

In the latest review (June 2012) 621 primary arthroplasties have been reviewed in detail at a mean follow-up of 13 years (10–15 years) [4]. A well maintained or improved bone stock or bone-cement interface was observed in 78.2 % of cases. No stem was "at risk" for loosening. Two stems fractured because of technical error – lack of proximal stem support by cement.

It must be appreciated that the beneficial radiographic changes, of the proximal femur or the bone-cement interface, may not be expected in all cases. It is inevitable that some of the changes are due to section of the femoral neck and some due to introduction of the intramedullary load-bearing construct. These changes may not be overcome if the load required, as governed by the patient's activity level, has not been reached. Declining function would be expected to have the same effect.

In some publications on the subject in would appear that the details of the surgical technique may not have been correctly interpreted.

References

1. Wroblewski BM, van der Rijt AJ. Intramedullary cancellous bone block to improve femoral stem fixation in Charnley low friction arthroplasty. J Bone Joint Surg (Br). 1984;66-B:639–44.
2. Wroblewski BM, Fleming PA, Hall RM, Siney PD. Stem fixation in the Charnley low friction arthroplasty in young patients using an intramedullary bone block. J Bone Joint Surg (Br). 1998;80-B:273–8.
3. Wroblewski BM, Siney PD, Fleming PA. Triple taper polished cemented stem in total hip arthroplasty: rationale for the design, surgical technique, and 7 years of clinical experience. J Arthroplasty. 2001;16(8 Suppl 1):37–41.
4. Purbach B, Kay PR, Siney PD, Fleming PA, Wroblewski BM. The C-Stem in clinical practice: fifteen-year follow-up of a triple tapered polished cemented stem. J Arthroplasty. 2013;28(8):1367–71.

Part V
The Cup

Chapter 27
The Charnley Acetabular Cup

It is hoped that the whole range of sockets in time will be replaced by the one single type and size of pressure injection design which can be cut down to suit all sizes of adult acetabulum. The very small (35 mm diameter) socket with offset bore will be the only exception. (1979).

A surgeon, not familiar with either the history of evolution of the cup design or the method of measurement may find the statement "… *"one type and size which can be cut down to suit all sizes…."* baffling.

Evolution of the design of the Charnley cup has received little attention. The reason for this is by no means clear. Was it the introduction of the new plastic, ultra high molecular weight polyethylene for its manufacture, was it the small 22.225 mm diameter head of the femoral component, the well documented details of surgical technique, or merely the spectacular clinical success of the operation? Wear of the cup presented much later. Design, probably interpreted as "size," was merely a side issue. The original, scalloped edge design, which has been adopted as the logo both of the John Charnley Trust and the John Charnley Research Institute, was followed by the flanged pressure injection cup (PIJ), and then the ogee-flanged cup. The changes had a purpose – to give stability of the cup at the trial and to improve containment and pressure of cement injection at the final insertion. Surgeons who did not follow the evolution of the cup design have missed its importance in clinical practice.

The Bore of the Cup

In the manufacture of the cup the bore is central. The depth of the bore is that of the radius of the femoral component with a 2 mm parallel lead-in section (Fig. 27.1).

© Springer International Publishing Switzerland 2016
B.M. Wroblewski et al., *Charnley Low-Frictional Torque Arthroplasty of the Hip: Practice and Results*, DOI 10.1007/978-3-319-21320-0_27

Fig. 27.1 Diagram of the
bore of the cup. The depth
of the bore is equal to the
radius of the head of the
femoral component with a
2 mm parallel lead-in
section

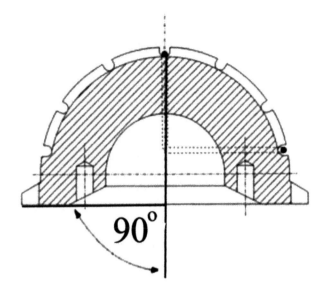

The Original UHMWPE Scalloped Cup Design

The hemispherical cup with a scalloped edge was the standard design (Figs. 27.2
and 27.3). Its face was chamfered. It could be used right or left, anterior or posterior,
as long as the wire marker was in the coronal plane. At insertion the cup was held in
a pair of stout artery forceps; the self-ejecting cup holder came later. Since the cup
dimensions could not be altered, except by choosing a small or a large size, the measurements were taken from the scalloped margin and not from the cup wall. The two
sizes available were 50 mm and 47 mm diameter (*"for the longest life of a socket the
optimum size of the femoral head will be half that of the external diameter of the
socket"*). The cup did fit within the prepared acetabular cavity since the preparation
with the reamers was towards the opposite shoulder (Figs. 27.4, 27.5, 27.6 and 27.7).

The Flanged Cup: Pressure Injection Cup (PIJ)
(Figs. 27.8 and 27.9)

With preparation of the acetabulum in the transverse direction (Nov 1970) the superior margin of the acetabulum was no longer covered by the rim of the cup allowing
escape of the cement. The solution was … *"to design the cup with an oval flange
inclined at 45° away from the face."* Thus the flanged PIJ cup was designed. Since
the bore of the cup was symmetrical the cup could be used right and left – as long
as the PIJ flange was always superiorly. The trimming of the flange to size and the
shape of the acetabular cavity improved the fit, stability of the cup at insertion, as
well as cement injection.

Figs. 27.2 and 27.3 The
original, scalloped edge,
Charnley cup, front and
back views

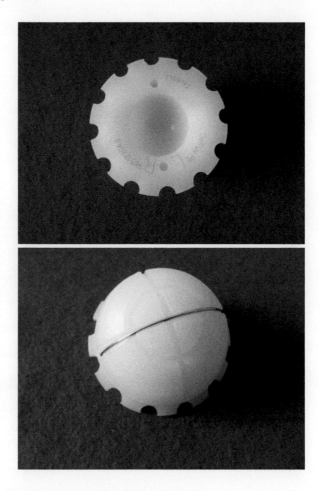

The Long Posterior Wall Cup (LPW) (Fig. 27.10)

The concept of the LPW cup is best understood if the method of cup machining
from a solid hemisphere is taken into account. Any cup is essentially a hemisphere
with a flat face. The central bore will accept the head of the femoral component, the
face is chamfered to put off the moment of impingement of the neck of the stem. If
only three quarters of the circumference is chamfered the remaining part of the flat
face forms an extension of the bore – the long posterior wall. Such a cup must not
be placed in anteversion "… *because this would increase the projection of the posterior wall and could cause impingement against the back of the neck in a fully
extended position of the hip*." It was introduced in May 1972 probably to placate
some surgeons who experienced a high incidence of post-operative dislocation
using a posterior approach to the hip joint.

Introduction of the long posterior wall cup (LPW) did not allow the use of an
asymmetric flange; the cup had to be for either right or left side. To overcome the

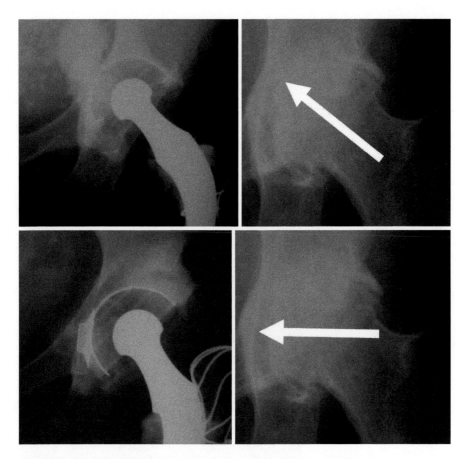

Figs. 27.4, 27.5, 27.6 and 27.7 Original technique of reaming the acetabulum

problem, the flange was extended to the opposite margin of the cup thus allowing a single design, but trimming of the inferior margin of the flange was now essential.

When the trimmable flange was introduced the scalloped edge had to be abandoned: the cup and the flange were machined from solid as a single unit. The trimmable flange was now considered as the extension of the cup size allowing "*the range of sizes*", while the body of the cup remained unchanged hence "*…one type and size which can be cut down to suit all sizes…*" The cutting down referred to the flange and not the cup.

The Ogee Flanged Cup (Fig. 27.11)

<u>Ogee</u>: an architectural term showing in a section a double continuous curve.

The standard symmetrical flange, when trimmed for size and shape of the acetabulum, was designed for the purpose of containing and pressurising the cement.

Figs. 27.8 and 27.9 Acetabular cup with a flange, front and back views

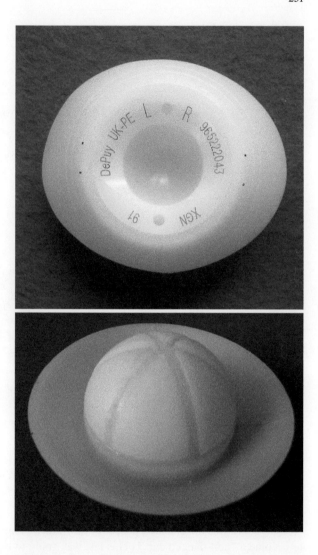

How successful it would prove to be in clinical application would take time, numbers and follow-up. Two further problems had to be addressed: machining from solid was expensive and time consuming. The symmetrical flange left the posterior aspect of the acetabulum uncovered thus reducing the area of bone-cement contact. The problems were addressed by changing the design of the flange and its method of manufacture. The flange was injection moulded separately with the posterior part now flaring out, while its anterior part remained turned medially = the ogee flange. This was the final design made by Sir John Charnley (Mr John Older – working very closely with Sir John – holds the longest clinical experience with this design as well as the history of the evolution of the concept). Experimental evaluation simulating clinical application has been published (Shelley 1988) [1].

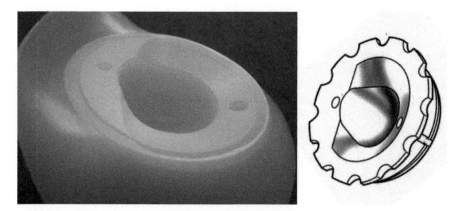

Fig. 27.10   Long posterior wall cup

Fig. 27.11   Angle-bore cup
with ogee flange and
trimmable aid

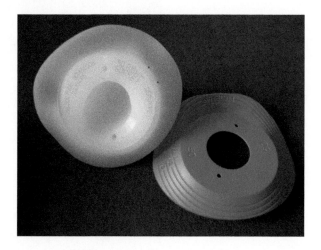

    Later there was the question posed: of how much flange had to be removed for it
to become a "non-flanged cup." (This last was going to be a difficult subject in the
long-term follow-up and may never be answered to everybody's satisfaction).

The 35 mm Diameter Offset-Bore Cup (Fig. 27.12)

The design was dictated by the clinical need of a smaller diameter cup as in some
cases of hip dysplasia or chronic juvenile rheumatoid arthritis. Reducing the
diameter to 35 mm, but still maintaining the central position of the bore would
give just 6 mm wall thickness. This was considered insufficient, 6 mm would not

Fig. 27.12 Radiograph of
a 35 mm offset-bore cup

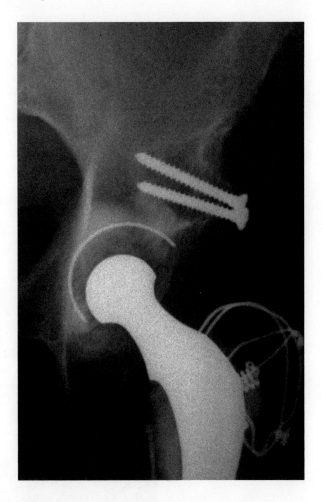

be adequate to resist the deformation of the thin UHMWPE shell under load.
With a penetration rate of 0.2 mm/year as an average in young active patients and
0.6 mm/year in extreme cases, even a 10 year expectancy was not considered
sufficient. There was also the question of low-frictional torque principle: the 35:
22.225 cup: head ratio would be no more than 1.6:1 at best probably too far
removed from the ideal 2:1 for metal on UHMWPE articulation [2]. Placing the
bore off-centre would increase the wall thickness in one sector of the cup, which
now always had to be implanted in the correct position – the thickest part superiorly – and would go some way to maintaining the 2:1 cup to head diameter
ratio. The offset-bore cup design does not have the parallel 2 mm leading-in
section.

The benefits of the design were obvious – the long-term benefits were to come.
They are presented in later in this volume.

The Wire Marker

To enable the wear of the socket to be measured over a period of many years in the human body, a semicircular radiographic marker was attached to the outer surface of all HMWP sockets used in this unit since early 1963. When performing the operation the plane of this wire marker is placed close to the coronal plane of the pelvis using a special holder to orientate the socket. A check on the reproducibility ... found that measurements were remarkably insensitive to the variations in the centering of the X-ray tube ... without affecting measurements by a significant amount.

In a handful of the original LFAs the components were fixed with acrylic cement, without barium sulphate as the opacifier, and the cup without a wire marker. The problem was immediately obvious – only the stem is visible on the post-operative radiograph (Fig. 27.13).

A hemispherical wire marker, in the coronal plane of the cup, was added and Barium Sulphate was included as a separate pack with the cement. The ends of the

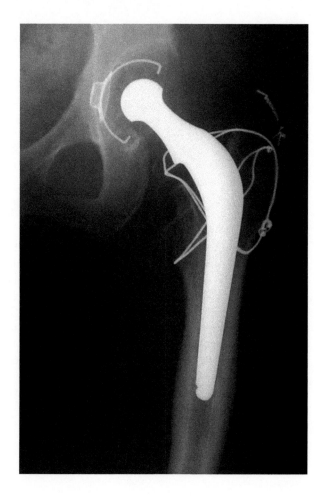

Fig. 27.13 Radiograph of early Charnley LFA showing cement without barium sulphate

Fig. 27.14 Wire marker to
measure wear the
UHMWPE cup – the
original version. (see
radiograph Fig. 27.4)

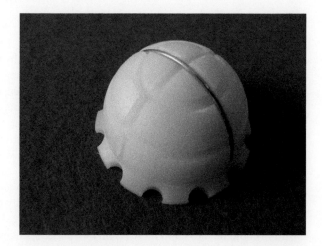

Fig. 27.15 Wire marker to
distinguish the long
posterior wall cup – note
the semicircular shape
without anchoring ends.
(see radiograph Fig. 27.6)

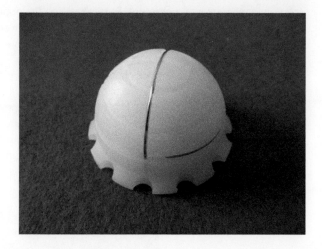

wire marker were bent over and clipped into locating holes at the rim of the cup to
keep the marker in place (Fig. 27.14).

The long posterior wall (LPW) cup, its radiographic appearance and its role in
addressing the post-operative dislocation rate still further, demanded a distinguish-
ing marker. The wire marker was made to conform to a full hemisphere of the cup
with the free end being flush with the face of the cup. This allowed an easy distinction between the standard cup with the scalloped edge and the LPW cup, whether
the latter was standard with scalloped edge, flanged or ogee flanged design
(Fig. 27.15).

The wire marker serves to indicate the position of the cup and the depth of cup
penetration when measuring the head – wire marker distance.

The Version Wire Marker

The design was a planned answer to a problem discussed by the late Professor Sir John Charnley and the late Professor Maurice Muller of Berne. This took place at the end of 1969 between operating sessions. The question posed was: how to measure the anteversion of the cup on a single antero-posterior radiograph? The single coronal wear marker was not suitable for the purpose. Christiansen and Charnley [3] commented on the subject pointing out that anteversion or retroversion of some 15° would be needed to affect the distance between the head and the wear wire marker as seen on radiographs.

Clearly the wear marker was not sensitive enough to measure version of the cup. In any degree of version the cup marker "moved" initially closely to the plane of the X-ray beam, it was only when the marker moved across the X-ray beam that its position could be measured more readily. Another semicircular wire attached to the rim of the cup, anteriorly, could be used to measure anteversion [4]. With anteversion of the cup the new marker would appear closer to the wear marker (Fig. 27.16) giving it an appearance of a crescent. In retroversion the opposite would be seen – the anteversion marker would be further away from the wear marker (Figs. 27.17, 27.18 and 27.19). The new design has its disadvantages. As the position of the wear marker is insensitive to changes of version of the cup, so the position of the version marker is very sensitive to that change. As the cup is placed into anteversion the marker moves across the X-ray beam and its position is further exaggerated on its projection onto the X-ray plate. It is also sensitive to position of the X-ray beam. Attempts to standardise the centre of the beam on a constant point – e.g. femoral artery in the groin, proved cumbersome and time consuming. The value of the anteversion marker has been established over the years of clinical practice: a retroverted cup is readily seen on the post-operative radiograph as is excessive anteversion. At

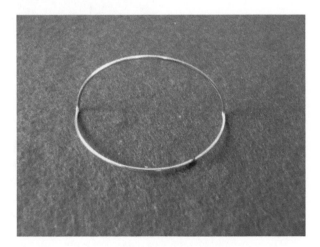

Fig. 27.16 Anteversion wire marker by itself

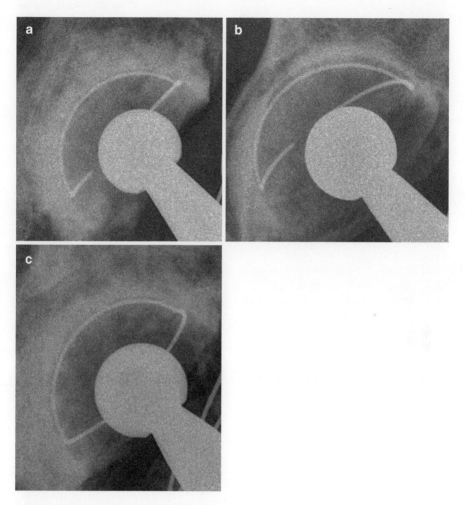

Figs. 27.17, 27.18 and 27.19 Anteversion wire marker to illustrate appearances with the cup in: – (**a**) neutral (**b**) anteverted (**c**) retroverted position

follow-up it is the change of configuration of the two markers, now attached to the cup as two continuous semicircles at right angles to each other, which offers important information in the study of post-operative dislocations and can be used as an indication of cup migration. A more detailed explanation of the radiographic appearances in relation to cup orientation can be taken from the DePuy International product information chart. The anteversion wire marker is a standard item.

(The circumferential wire marker in the plane of the face of the cup does not distinguish the version from an antero-posterior radiograph).

References

1. Shelley P, Wroblewski BM. Socket design and cement pressurisation in the Charnley low-friction arthroplasty. J Bone Joint Surg (Br). 1988;70-B:358–63.
2. Charnley J, Kamangar A, Longfield MD. The optimum size of prosthetic heads in relation to the wear of plastic sockets in total replacement of the hip. Med Biol Eng. 1969;7:31–9.
3. Christiansen C, Charnley J. The accuracy of radiological measurements of wear of the plastic hip socket in vivo. Internal publication No 21. 1969. Centre for Hip Surgery, Wrightington Hospital.
4. Wroblewski BM. Revision surgery in total hip arthroplasty. Berlin: Springer; 1990. p. 36–7.

Chapter 28
Bone-Cement Interface: The Cup: Radiographic Appearances

Demarcation on the radiographs is seen as a dark line between the radiopaque cement and the bone of the acetabulum. ... the width was measured on the radiographs ... and its distribution categorised into three zones I, II, or III. The radiographs were also scrutinised for bulk migration.

The complexity of this aspect of total hip arthroplasty was clearly documented by DeLee and Charnley [1]. A number of factors, either singly or a combination, affect the result. Design, materials, surgical technique, the method of component fixation, patient's activity level, the length of follow-up, wear and mechanical changes resulting, as well as tissue reaction to wear particles, radiographic appearances, clinical results, findings at revision surgery and the histology of the bone-cement interface, are some of the important issues.

Demarcation of the Cup

Radiographic appearances are best recorded using accepted terminology without any attempt to correlate them to, or combine them with, the clinical results. The DeLee – Charnley description and classification [1] is accepted as the standard. The hemisphere of the cup is divided into three segments: $I=45°$: $II=90°$: $III=45°$ (Fig. 28.1). Why this unequal division is by no means clear.

The description is clearly one of *"demarcation ... seen as a dark line between the radiopaque cement and the bone of the acetabulum."* Histological examination revealed a fibrous tissue layer between bone and cement. This layer varied in appearance. *"Thick layers of soft fibrous tissue ...frequently alternate with thin layers of dense fibrous tissue ... often the cement makes load-bearing contact with the underlying bone which closely resembles fibrocartilage.*

© Springer International Publishing Switzerland 2016
B.M. Wroblewski et al., *Charnley Low-Frictional Torque Arthroplasty of the Hip: Practice and Results*, DOI 10.1007/978-3-319-21320-0_28

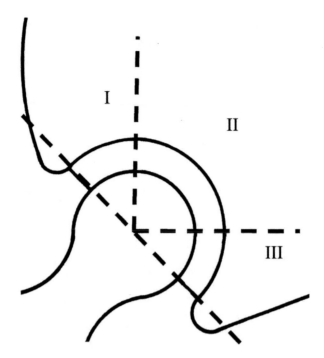

Fig. 28.1 Cup demarcation grading of DeLee and Charnley, showing division of hemisphere of acetabular bone-cement interface into zones, type I, II, III (Reproduced with permission from DeLee and Charnley [1])

The conclusion was:

- *"The vast majority with demarcation were symptomless."*
- *"… where demarcation was associated with migration … technical explanation or low grade sepsis was responsible."*
- *"better surgical technique may increase the number of cases showing no demarcation."*

Correlation Between Radiographic Appearances and Operative Findings [2]

This study was undertaken to establish the correlation between the radiographic appearances and the operative findings at the bone-cement interface of the cup of the Charnley LFA.

Method of Testing for Cup Loosening

The margin of the cup and the bone cement junction is exposed using Charnley gouges: This may include removal of the marginal osteophytes. The acetabulum retractor introduced into the margin of the obdurator foramen exposes the inferior margin of the cup where wear debris usually accumulates. The socket tester is screwed into one of the cup holder locating holes. Gentle rotating movement is applied to the tester while the bone-cement junction is observed. Movement, and at times fluid ejection, at the bone-cement interface is taken as evidence of cup loosening. (Extensive demarcation of the outer one third of the cup and gross wear allowing elastic deflection of the UHMWPE cup wall will produce a similar effect.) More than one area of the bone-cement junction must be examined.

Two hundred consecutive revisions were studied. This was a single surgeon series (BMW) examined independently by surgeon (JPH) without reference to the operative findings, until completion of the study.

Radiographic appearances were classified.

Type 0 = No demarcation.
Type 1 = Demarcation of outer 1/3
Type 2 = Demarcation of outer 1/3 and middle 1/3
Type 3 = Complete demarcation.
Type 4 = Cup migration (change of position on serial radiographs).

(Note: the hemisphere of cup-cement complex divided into three equal segments of 60° each, unlike DeLee) (Fig. 28.2).

The correlation between radiographic appearances and operative findings is shown in Tables 28.1, 28.2 and Fig. 28.3.

The conclusion was that all cups showing no demarcation were soundly fixed. If the demarcation involved the outer $^1/_3$ but was less than 1 mm, the cups were secure. However, if this was more than 1 mm, 18.5 % of cups were loose. As the demarcation extended to the outer $^2/_3$, 71 % of the cups were loose: 22 % if the demarcation was less than 1 mm, but 95 % if this was more than 1 mm. The corresponding findings with full cup demarcation was 94 %: 62.5 % if the demarcation was less than 1 mm and 100 % when this was greater than 1 mm.

If demarcation of the bone-cement interface be correlated with the incidence of cup loosening, then the ideal would be no demarcation at all or not more than the outer $^1/_3$ and less than 1 mm. **It is suggested that for practical purposes complete demarcation of the bone-cement interface measuring 1 mm or less is accepted as indicating a secure cup. More extensive demarcation must, therefore, indicate a loose cup.**

One year radiograph is useful in predicting long-term results. The findings in this study offer a good indicator for follow-up with good quality serial radiographs. It must be accepted, however, that clinical results do not reflect the mechanical state of the arthroplasty [4].

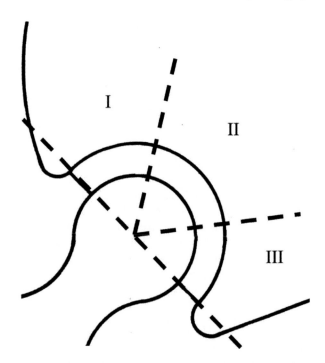

Fig. 28.2 Cup demarcation grading of Hodgkinson et al. showing division of hemisphere of acetabular bone-cement interface into equal zones, type I, II, III (Reproduced with permission from Hodgkinson et al. [2])

Table 28.1 Comparison of radiographic appearances and the operative findings

	Demarcation type				
	0	1	2	3	4
Number of cases	24	68	28	52	28
Number of loose cups	0	5	20	49	28
% Loose cups	0	7	71	94	100

Table 28.2 Correlation between width of demarcation of the bone-cement interface and the operative findings

Demarcation	Number of cups	Gap size at widest point (mm)	Sockets in each group	Firm cups	Loose cups (No)	Loose cups (%)
Type 1	68	<1	41	41	0	0
		>1	27	22	5	18.5
Type 2	28	<1	9	7	2	22.2
		>1	19	1	18	95
Type 3	52	<1	8	3	5	62.5
		>1	44	0	44	100

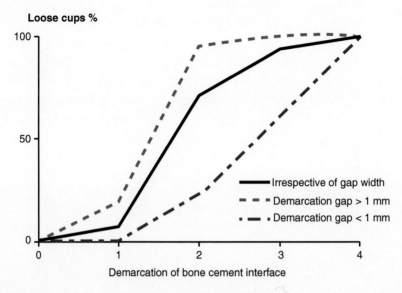

Fig. 28.3 Demarcation of the bone cement interface and the incidence of loose cups at revision surgery (Reproduced from Wroblewski [3])

References

1. DeLee JG, Charnley J. Radiological demarcation of cemented sockets in total hip replacement. Clin Orthop Relat Res. 1976;2:20–32.
2. Hodgkinson JP, Shelley P, Wroblewski BM. The correlation between the roentgenographic appearances and operative findings at the bone-cement junction of the socket in Charnley low-friction arthroplasties. Clin Orthop Relat Res. 1988;28:105–9.
3. Wroblewski BM. Revision surgery in total hip arthroplasty. London: Springer; 1990.
4. Wroblewski BM, Fleming PA, Siney PD. Charnley low-frictional torque arthroplasty of the hip. 20 to 30 year results. J Bone Joint Surg. 1999;81-B:427–30.

Chapter 29
The Effect of Cup Inclination on Contact Mechanics

In any design or method of cup fixation the one limiting factor is the space available within the variable quality of the acetabular bone stock. With the acrylic cement, having ensured the quality of bone-cement interface, the cup position/orientation can be adjusted within the polymerising cement mass.

With "cementless" techniques the room for manoeuvre is limited. The aim is to prepare the cavity to accept a press-fit symmetric cup into a predetermined position and orientation. This becomes more complex with increasing dimensions of hard on hard articulations and even more so when the need to preserve the femoral bone stock becomes the guiding principle.

Attempts to establish the "safe zone" for cup position and orientation gained priority [1].

With the Charnley technique the operative details were stated [2] and the long term results published [3].

The Effect of Cup Inclination and Wear on the Contact Mechanics and Cement Fixation [4]

An investigation was carried out to study the individual and combined influences of the cup inclination and penetration on contact mechanics and fixation using finite element analysis.

Results

On the initial bedding in of the metal head within the UHMWPE cup, the maximum contact pressure was reduced by 30 % and the bone-cement stress by 20 %.

© Springer International Publishing Switzerland 2016
B.M. Wroblewski et al., *Charnley Low-Frictional Torque Arthroplasty of the Hip: Practice and Results*, DOI 10.1007/978-3-319-21320-0_29

There was no further appreciable change at various depths of cup penetration up to 4 mm and the cup inclination up to 55°

Increasing the cup inclination to 65° together with cup penetration of 4 mm resulted in large increases of stress at the bone-cement.

Conclusion

The results confirm the original Charnley concept of design, materials and the method of component fixation. This is further confirmed by the published 30–40 year results. The information offers some indication as to the next stage of development in order to extend the successful results with LFTA still further.

References

1. Lewinnek GE, Lewis JL, Torr RR, Compere CL, Zimmerman JR. Dislocation after total hip replacement arthroplasties. J Bone Joint Surg (Am). 1978;60-A:217–20.
2. Charnley J. Low friction arthroplasty of the hip. Theory and practice. Berlin: Springer; 1979.
3. Wroblewski BM, Siney PD, Fleming PA. Charnley low-frictional torque arthroplasty. Follow-up for 30–40 years. J Bone Joint Surg (Br). 2009;91-B:447–50.
4. Xijin Hua, Wroblewski BM, Zhongmin Jin, Ling Wang. The effect of cup inclination and wear on the contact mechanics and cement fixation for ultra high molecular weight polyethylene total hip replacements. Med Eng Phys 2012;34:318–325.

Part VI
Wear

Chapter 30
Wear of the UHMWPE Cup

The failure, if it does eventually supervene, is to be expected from one, or both, of two possible causes:

"Tissue reaction to particles abraded from the bearing surface;" and Mechanical loosening of the cement bond in the bone. 1961.

The study of socket wear/creep and the resultant loosening is urgent, and at this stage may appear to be the one factor limiting the life of the arthroplasty. (1984).

Wear

Removal or transfer of material from contacting surfaces due to their relative movement under load. Wear can be measured by mass change, volume measurement or by the depth of the wear tracks. **The two inevitable consequences are shedding of wear products and change of the geometry of the articulation**.

Study of wear in THA is a complex task. It involves a number of closely related topics: materials, design, surgical technique as well as the consequences of wear be they mechanical or biological. It is therefore important that the whole topic is studied in the context of the principle of the design, clinical practice and the long term results.

Some repetition in the text is not only inevitable, but also essential to maintain the continuity.

The Information Gathered from the Teflon Era

It was during that period that the design of the components, *"the mechanical details of the technique became stabilised in the period 1959 to 1962 ..."* (1979)

© Springer International Publishing Switzerland 2016
B.M. Wroblewski et al., *Charnley Low-Frictional Torque Arthroplasty of the Hip: Practice and Results*, DOI 10.1007/978-3-319-21320-0_30

Sockets did not wear by enlargement … in all directions in a random fashion … plastic socket in the hip joint retains permanently a close fit against the spherical metal head.

… it would follow that the smallest volume of harmful particulate matter would be generated by using the smallest head which anatomical and mechanical considerations would permit.

… from consideration of the geometry and wear characteristics … the sphere should have a diameter not greater than half that of the external diameter of the socket.

… wear is related more to the grade of functional activity than to the weight of the subject.

… this material (wear debris) *is pumped … by every movement of the joint and eventually it starts to erode in the place of contact between the socket and its bed.*

In small amounts there seems nothing harmful in particles of PTFE since we have many instances of this material in the human tissues where it has become sealed off and …calcified over periods of seven and eight years.

Measurements of Wear: Early Stages [1, 2]

The question of methods of wear measurement was tackled later – when UHMWPE was used routinely and fixed with acrylic cement.

The earliest detailed report stated: *"To calculate the amount of wear, the narrowest measurement of the head – wire wear marker distance in the weight-bearing area is subtracted from the widest measurement in the non-weight-bearing zone, and the difference is then divided by 2." "…without the need to correct for magnification"* (1973) [1].

Charnley argued against the criticism of the method … *"…the criticism would be accurate in only two extreme cases."* In all subsequent studies *"…measurements were corrected for magnification by a factor from comparing the diameter of the femoral head on the radiograph with its known diameter of 22.225 mm"* (1975) [2].

Charnley and Halley [2] speculated further …*"…it is thought that more than 5 mm wear might cause impingement of the neck of the prosthesis against the inner rim of the socket and cause loosening of the cement-bone bond of the acetabulum"*

"From these studies (1973 and 1975) the average rate of wear (UHMWPE cup) was accepted as 0.15 mm/year."

Although the study of wear of the UHMWPE cup was of interest from the time the material was introduced into clinical practice, its importance became more obvious with increasing follow-up. There was a need for an easy, clinically useful and relatively accurate method of measurement that could take advantage of the availability of serial radiographs. It is for that purpose that the radiographic wire marker was added to the cup.

The study by Griffith, Seidenstein, Williams and Charnley [3] has served the purpose well. The findings are summarised here:

– Radiographs of 491 LFAs were examined.
– Mean follow-up 8.3 years (7–9 years).

- Mean penetration rate was 0.07 mm/year.
- Total penetration for the whole group was 0.59 mm.
- 63.5 % showed a total penetration of less than 0.5 mm and a rate less than 0.06 mm/year.
- In 4 % total penetration was 1.9 mm (1.5–2.8 mm) and a penetration rate of 0.24 mm/year.
- Males had a higher penetration rate than females, as did the younger patients.
- There was no clear correlation between body mass and wear.
- Study of activity level and wear has shown that: unless function is grade 6 (normal) for several years, heavy wear does not occur.

These results should be accepted as baseline for future studies with increasing follow-up.

Longer follow-up, increasing number of revisions and availability of explanted components stimulated further research, and developments, into all aspects of wear of the UHMWPE cup in the Charnley LFA. Although some of the investigations were undertaken mainly for scientific reasons – pure research – most of them were directed towards establishing the causes of cup wear and loosening in an attempt to reduce, if not eliminate wear as the one factor limiting the life of the arthroplasty.

(The frequently quoted method attributed to Livermore et al. [4] is not original; it is based on the Griffith et al. study [3] as is clearly stated by the authors. "The radiographic measurements were made as described by Griffith et al.").

References

1. Charnley J, Cupic Z. The nine and ten year results of the low-friction arthroplasty of the hip. Clin Orthop Relat Res. 1973;85:9–25.
2. Charnley J, Halley DK. Rate of wear in total hip replacement. Clin Orthop Relat Res. 1975;112:170–9.
3. Griffith MJ, Seidenstein MK, Williams D, Charnley J. Socket wear in Charnley low-friction arthroplasty of the hip. Clin Orthop Relat Res. 1978;137:37–47.
4. Livermore J, Ilstrup D, Morrey B. Effect of femoral head size on wear of polyethylene acetabular component. J Bone Joint Surg (Am). 1990;72-A:518–28.

Chapter 31
The Principle of Low Frictional Torque in Clinical Practice

The theme of this work is the application of the engineering theory of frictional torque to total hip replacement.

Can the benefit of the low-frictional torque be demonstrated in the long-term results of the Charnley LFA?

The statement, in Charnley's final definitive volume: "Low friction arthroplasty of the hip. Theory and Practice" summarizes the concept and its application in clinical practice. The smallest, practically acceptable diameter head of the stainless steel femoral component, articulating with a thick-walled UHMWPE cup. This would encourage movement, preferentially at the level of the articulation rather than at the bone-cement interface, thus reducing the likelihood of cup loosening. Why has this basic principle not been generally recognised and accepted in clinical practice? Was the use of large diameter heads driven by fear of post-operative dislocation? Was the use of hard on hard articulations dictated by the belief that tissue reaction to UHMWPE wear particles is responsible for component loosening? It is probably correct to suggest that even Charnley had some doubts as to the importance of low-frictional torque principle as applied in clinical practice.

"*The property of the low-frictional resistance in the artificial joint does not appear to reveal itself in the clinical results as a matter of such importance as I had originally imagined.*" (1966) UHMWPE had already been routinely used for 4 years, the principles of the design, materials and the details of the surgical technique were established. A total of 1321 LFAs had been implanted and none have been revised for loosening of the cup, the stem or fracture of the stem. Clinical success, absence of revisions and lack of reports of other designs to allow any comparison, probably prompted Charnley's statement. It was two further years and 1180 LFAs before the first revision, for the above mentioned complications, had to be carried out.

Anderson and colleagues (1972) questioned the significance of low-frictional torque as a contributor to the preservation of the bone-cement interface. They compared torsional moments needed to loosen cemented Charnley and metal on metal McKee design cups. They concluded that the torsional moments were

© Springer International Publishing Switzerland 2016
253
B.M. Wroblewski et al., *Charnley Low-Frictional Torque Arthroplasty of the Hip:
Practice and Results*, DOI 10.1007/978-3-319-21320-0_31

from 4 to more than 25 times higher than the frictional moments measured and, therefore, unlikely to contribute top cup loosening. Charnley argued "...*that if the demarcation of the cemented socket from the adjacent cancellous bone is present, the avoidance of high frictional torque might permit such a socket to function for many years than would be the case if the high frictional torque were present.*" (1978)

In 1981/1982 Charnley reviewed the longest follow-up results available. He pointed out that "...*gross demarcation, together with migration, affected a total of 25 % of sockets, though at the time of the review none of these patients showed any clinical defect. Given time and function 25 % of sockets were expected to fail by migration.*" But "*where severe demarcation was present, the fact that the migration of the socket had not progressed to clinical failure was attributed to the delaying action of the low-frictional torque using small diameter prosthetic heads.*"

Charnley recognised aseptic loosening of the cemented UHMWPE cup as occurring at two levels: radiological and clinical. Radiological failure was described as: "... *the operations judged on clinical grounds are still successful, but the radiological appearances indicate ...that sooner or later the clinical failure must follow.*" Clinical failure: "... *pain returns, the early excellent function following the operation is lost and re-operation may be necessary.*"

It is probably correct to suggest that misunderstandings and even confusion regarding interpretation of results of various total hip joint designs and methods, could have been avoided, if a strict distinction was made between clinical results and radiographic appearances.

Freedom from pain is due to the neuropathic nature of the arthroplasty – subject to correct patient selection and sound fixation of the components. Patients' activity level is a reflection of patient selection for the operation. Clinical results do not reflect the mechanical state of the arthroplasty; loose and even migrating components are not necessarily symptomatic [1].

Ma and colleagues [2] studied frictional torque both in resurfacing and conventional hip replacements with cemented UHMWPE cups. They concluded that frictional torque was proportional to the diameter of the head of the femoral component; it was lowered as the thickness of the cup was increased.

Ritter and colleagues [3] compared the results of 67 Mueller arthroplasties (32 mm head, 50 mm cup diameter) with 300 Charnley arthroplasties (22 mm head, 44 mm cup diameter) at a minimum follow-up of 7 years. The incidence of cup loosening was 15 % compared with 4 %; survivorship at 5 years was 87 % compared with 94 %, and at 7 years 70 % compared with 86 % – were all in favour of the Charnley design.

When Morrey and colleagues [4] examined the correlation between the head size and acetabular revisions in 6128 arthroplasties, they concluded that "... although friction increases with the size of the femoral head theoretically, it remains significantly low that the bone-cement interface is not at risk". (The author's statement: "friction increase with the size of the femoral head" is not correct: frictional torque increases with the size of the femoral head, friction does not).

Radiolucent lines were more frequent with the 32 mm diameter head: 29 % as opposed to 15 % with the 22 mm diameter head. Even though the 32 mm head design was introduced after 5 years experience had been accumulated with the cementing of the 22 mm diameter heads, the incidence of aseptic cup loosening was still higher with the 32 mm diameter head: 6.8 % as compared with 2–3 % with the Charnley design. Similar experience was reported by Frankel et al. [5] "… three zone demarcation of the acetabular bone-cement was 56 % of the 32 mm group as compared with 5 % of the 22 mm group". Their conclusion was that "… these results emphasise the adverse affects of large femoral head prostheses on the bone-cement interface and underline the need for alternative methods of fixation". The authors make no suggestion as to what alternative methods of fixation could be used or how they would "circumvent the adverse effects of large head diameters."

Mai and colleagues [6] examined the contribution of frictional torque to loosening in Tharies hip replacements. The conclusions, based on 1970 cases with a follow-up to 16 years, did not support their suggestion that larger heads performed better. With an overall revision rate of 47.10 % there was no difference in the results whether the head diameter was small, medium or large (23.5 %, 23.5 % and 26.5 % revision rate). Their explanation was that "polyethylene wear has a greater effect on the durability of fixation of the implant than frictional torque does."

Published evidence supports the concept of low-frictional torque as the principle in total hip arthroplasty. The reasons for failure to implement this in clinical practice is by no means clear.

It was clearly essential to examine whether the benefit of the low-frictional torque could be demonstrated in the long-term results of the Charnley hip replacement, and, if so, what is the level of that benefit?

Low Frictional Torque in the Charnley Total Hip Arthroplasty

What Is the Benefit of the Low-Frictional Torque in Clinical Practice?

Theoretical considerations indicate that if the diameter of the head of the femoral component remains constant then any benefit of low-frictional torque would be proportional to the difference in the external radii of the cups, and would be expected to remain at comparable depths of cup penetration. In an attempt to answer the question we reviewed the information collected on the 1016 patients, mean age 41 years (15–50) 1332 LFAs with a follow-up to 40 years [7].

Wear of the cup was measured as penetration according to Griffith et al. [8] radiographic cup loosening as suggested by Hodgkinson et al. [9].

We compared the differences in the incidence of cup loosening between the cup sizes: 40 and 43 mm diameter at comparable depths of cup penetration.

The results are shown in Tables 31.1, 31.2 and Fig. 31.1.

Table 31.1 Demographic details

Cup diameter (mm)	40	43
Number of LFAs	453	879
Males	37	369
Females	301	309
Age years – mean (range)	40.3 (15–50)	41.7 (20–50)
Follow-up years – mean (range)	17 (1–35)	16.2 (1–37)
Cup loosening – no (%)	121 (26.7)	187 (21.3)

Table 31.2 Cup penetration and loosening

Cup penetration (mm)	Cup size (mm)	Number	Cup loosening Number	%
0	40	8	0	0
	43	21	0	0
<= 1	40	222	21	9.5
	43	438	35	8.0
<= 2	40	90	34	37.8
	43	169	49	29.0
<= 3	40	78	35	44.9
	43	128	45	35.2
<= 4	40	36	18	50.0
	43	52	21	40.4
>4	40	19	13	68.4
	43	71	37	52.1

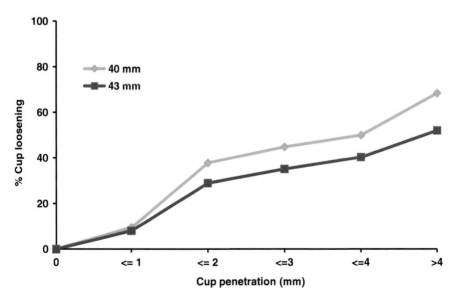

Fig. 31.1 Incidence of cup loosening between the cup sizes: 40 and 43 mm diameter at comparable depths of cup penetration

Interpretation of Results

When interpreting the results the thickness of the cement mantle is not taken into account. Measurement of the cement layer, in various areas, and the depth of penetration into cancellous bone, with any degree of accuracy is a daunting task. Whether this would contribute any valuable information is debatable. Excluding the cement layer reduces the external diameter of the cup-cement construct and thus presents the smallest and the least advantageous cup-head diameter ratios.

It is accepted that a number of factors are involved in the rate of cup penetration. Some of them may also have an effect on the integrity of the bone-cement interface. It is because of the complexity of the concept as applied to clinical practice that we have limited the interpretation to comparing the **incidence of aseptic cup loosening at a comparable depth of cup penetration, irrespective of the penetration rate**.

With the Charnley design the cup-head diameter ratio is 1.8:1 for the 40 mm cup and 1.9:1 for the 43 mm cup. A cement layer of only 2 mm would increase this ratio to 2:1 and bring this to the advantageous ratio as suggested by Charnley et al. [10]. The difference in the external diameters of the two cup sizes is 7–7.5 %. There were 29 cups with no measurable wear; the follow-up was 11–12 years; none were radiologically loose. Increasing depth of cup penetration was reflected in the difference in the incidence of aseptic cup loosening between the two cup sizes. This was 1.5 % at 1 mm, 8.8 % at 2 mm reaching 9.7–9.6 % at 3 and 4 mm penetration respectively, always in favour of the 43 mm diameter cup and close to the predicted values. Cup wear and loosening are processes. The results of that process are recorded at intervals imposed by the frequency of follow-up. It is the consistency of the pattern in the incidence of cup loosening for the two cup sizes that supports the original supposition. It can be argued that the difference is not particularly great. The magnitude of the difference is a reflection of the cup diameters used in clinical practice over a 45 year period. Size of the acetabular cavity is the factor limiting the ultimate diameter of the cup that can be used in any particular case.

With a total penetration above 4 mm impingement of the neck on the rim of the cup becomes the very potent mechanism of cup loosening [11].

Conclusion

Low frictional torque principle is an important factor in the design and practice of total hip arthroplasty. The benefit is reflected in the long-term results; the greater the cup-head diameter ratio the lower the incidence of aseptic cup loosening. The level of that benefit, expressed as a percentage, is proportional to the difference of the cup-head diameter ratios at comparable depths of cup penetration – up to 4 mm total penetration. When penetration exceeds 4 mm, impingement of the neck of the stem on the rim of the cup becomes the major factor leading to cup loosening.

The findings give supporting evidence to the importance of low frictional torque in the Charnley design. They also confirm that cup loosening is a mechanical and not a biological process.

References

1. Wroblewski BM, Fleming PA, Siney PD. Charnley low-frictional torque arthroplasty of the hip. 20 to 30 year results. J Bone Joint Surg. 1999;81-B:427–30.
2. Ma SM, Kabo JM, Amstutz HC. Frictional torque in surface and conventional hip replacement. J Bone Joint Surg Am. 1983;65-A:366–70.
3. Ritter MA, Stringer EA, Littrell DA, Williams JG. Correlation of prosthetic femoral head size and/or design with longevity of total hip arthroplasty. Clin Orthop. 1983;176:252–7.
4. Morrey BF, Ilstrup D. Size of the femoral head and acetabular revision in total hip replacement arthroplasty. J Bone Joint Surg Am. 1989;71-A:50–5.
5. Frankel A, Balderston RA, Booth RE, Rothman RH. Radiographic demarcation of the acetabular bone-cement interface: the effect of femoral head size. J Arthroplasty. 1990;5(Suppl):S1–3.
6. Mai MT, Schmalzried TP, Dorey J, Campbell PA, Amstutz HC. The contribution of frictional torque to loosening at the cement-bone interface in Tharies hip replacements. J Bone Joint Surg Am. 1996;78-A:505–11.
7. Wroblewski BM, Siney PD, Fleming PA. The principle of low frictional torque in the Charnley total hip replacement. J Bone Joint Surg. 2009;91-B:855–8.
8. Griffith MJ, Seidenstein MK, Williams D, Charnley J. Socket wear in Charnley low-friction arthroplasty of the hip. Clin Orthop. 1978;137:37.
9. Hodgkinson JP, Shelley P, Wroblewski BM. The correlation between roentgenographic appearances and operative findings at the bone-cement junction of the socket in the Charnley low-friction arthroplasties. Clin Orthop Relat Res. 1998;228:105–9.
10. Charnley J, Kamangar A, Longfield MD. The optimum size of prosthetic heads in relation to the wear of plastic sockets in total replacement of the hip. Med Biol Eng. 1969;7:31–9.
11. Wroblewski BM, Siney PD, Fleming PA. Effect of reduced diameter neck stem on the incidence of radiographic cup loosening and revisions in Charnley low-frictional torque arthroplasty. J Arthroplast. 2009;24:10–4.

Chapter 32
Comparison of Direct and Radiographic Wear Measurements

The study by Griffith et al. [1] has established the method of wear measurement of the UHMWPE on serial radiographs. It was essential that the results of the method were validated by comparison with measurements taken directly from explanted cups.

The Study

Acrylic casts (Fig. 32.1) and the shadowgraph technique (Fig. 32.2) were used to compare the real penetration of the cup with measurements taken from pre-revision radiographs. Twenty two paired observations were compared [2].

- The mean real (shadowgraph) penetration rate was 0.19 mm/year (0.017–0.52 mm/year) compared with 0.21 mm/year (0–0.41 mm/year) as measured on radiographs (Fig. 32.3).
- When the total penetration was less than 2 mm radiographs overestimated the rate.
- When the total penetration was more than 2 mm radiographs underestimated the rate.
- The overall correlation between the two methods was highly significant ($p < 0.001$) supporting the value of the radiographic method.
- Erosion of the margin of the cup bore was interpreted as evidence of impingement of the neck of the stem on the rim and a potent cause of cup loosening.
- With the 12.5 mm diameter neck the probability of impingement was estimated to occur once the depth of penetration of 0.4–0.56 mm had been reached.
- Theoretical model studies indicated that reducing the diameter of the neck of the Charnley stem from 12.5 to 10 mm would delay impingement and reduce the incidence of aseptic cup loosening by the equivalent of 3 mm of cup penetration (Fig. 32.4).

© Springer International Publishing Switzerland 2016
B.M. Wroblewski et al., *Charnley Low-Frictional Torque Arthroplasty of the Hip: Practice and Results*, DOI 10.1007/978-3-319-21320-0_32

Fig. 32.1 Acrylic cast used to measure the real penetration of the cup

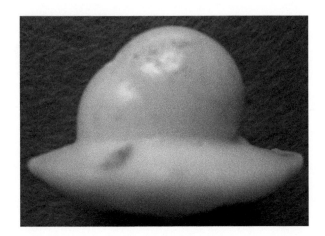

Fig. 32.2 Shadowgraph technique used to measure the penetration of the cup (Reproduced with permission and copyright © of the British Editorial Society of Bone and Joint Surgery from Wroblewski [2])

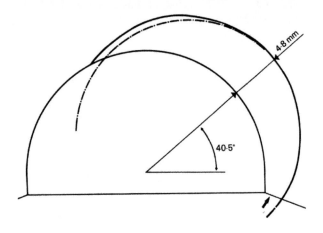

Fig. 32.3 Depth of cup penetration: Correlation between radiographic and acrylic cast measurements (Reproduced with permission and copyright © of the British Editorial Society of Bone and Joint Surgery from Wroblewski [2])

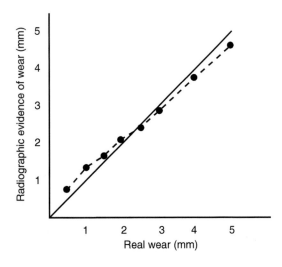

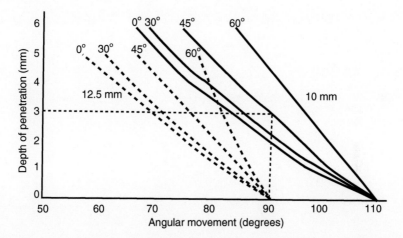

Fig. 32.4 Theoretical model studies indicated that reducing the diameter of the neck of the Charnley stem from 12.5 to 10 mm would delay impingement and reduce the incidence of aseptic cup loosening by the equivalent of 3 mm of cup penetration (Reproduced with permission and copyright © of the British Editorial Society of Bone and Joint Surgery from Wroblewski [2])

Hall et al. (1995) [3] measured wear in 28 explanted Charnley cups. They concluded that the "shadowgraph technique provided the most suitable method of measuring the dimensional changes in the retrieved sockets due to the relative ease of use."

References

1. Griffith MJ, Seidenstein MK, Williams D, Charnley J. Socket wear in the Charnley low-friction arthroplasty of the hip. Clin Orthop Relat Res. 1978;137:37–47.
2. Wroblewski BM. Direction and rate of socket wear in Charnley low-friction arthroplasty. J Bone Joint Surg (Br). 1985;67-B:757–61.
3. Hall RM, Unsworth A, Craig PS, Hardaker C, Siney P, Wroblewski BM. Measurement of wear in retrieved acetabular sockets. Proc Inst Mech Eng H. 1995;209(4):233–42.

Chapter 33
Penetration of UHMWPE Cup: Wear or Creep

<u>Creep:</u> Continuous deformation of material when subjected to stress over an extended period.

Aware of the possibility of creep of the UHMWPE cup, when under load in the human body, Charnley set up an experiment. Cemented cup was loaded through 22.225 mm diameter stainless steel head. The load was approximately one body mass; in the early 1960s this was taken to be approximately 76 kg. Displacement of the head into the cup – over many years, was micrometers only. It occurred early and did not progress with time (Fig. 33.1).

If creep did occur to any extent then "displaced" plastic would either heap up at the margin of the loaded area or be compressed into the subsurface of the contact area. No such changes were found. Creep, as a contribution to volumetric change, was considered not to be important. Dimensional changes were considered to be primarily due to wear.

Rose and colleagues 1980 [1] studied total prostheses of the Charnley – Mueller design by total joint simulation for the equivalent of 1 year of use using the "recovery of debris" method. They concluded that "… wear accounted for only small fractions (between 1 % and 30 %) of the dimensional changes", and that "… most of the changes previously ascribed to wear, were in fact due to creep or plastic flow." They did not consider that "… dimensional changes due to wear will be large enough to impair mechanical function." "Thus, the chief clinical question is the biological effect of the debris and not the mechanical problems due to dimensional changes." [1].

The reasoning behind the conclusion is not entirely clear. The authors claim that dimensional changes are primarily due to creep, whilst wear accounts for only 1–30 % of these changes, and yet, the main problem they consider is due to "biological effects of the debris."

– Isaac et al. [2] examined 87 explanted Charnley cups. The average follow-up was 8.75 years (0.2–18.6 years) and mean age at surgery of 55 years (19–73 years).

© Springer International Publishing Switzerland 2016
B.M. Wroblewski et al., *Charnley Low-Frictional Torque Arthroplasty of the Hip: Practice and Results*, DOI 10.1007/978-3-319-21320-0_33

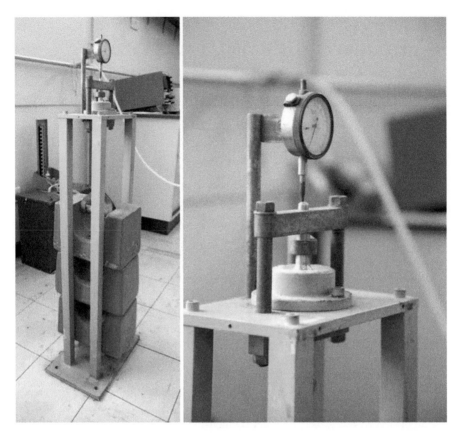

Fig. 33.1 Long term testing of UHMWPE cup under a constant load of 76 kg in an attempt to measure creep

Penetration was measured using shadowgraphs of acrylic casts. The results of this very detailed study did not resolve the question posed in the title: wear, creep or degradation? The conclusion was that the initial, relatively rapid irrecoverable deformation process was followed by a steady, much lower and decreasing penetration rate associated with wear. There was no evidence to suggest that the method of sterilisation – chemical (formalin soak) or gamma irradiation in air, had any effect on wear that could distinguish the two methods.

- Hall et al. [3] used a shadowgraph technique to examine 129 Charnley cups retrieved at revisions. Patients' mean age at surgery was 56 years (12–78 years) and mean time to revision was 10.7 years (0.75–22 years). The conclusion was that creep component was not a significant proportion of the overall change in the inner bore. The findings also indicated that ingress of cement particles into the articulation occur immediately after the primary operation [3].
- In prospective clinical and joint simulator studies of alumina ceramic on chemically cross-linked polyethylene, the UHMWPE cups showed relatively high rates

of penetration in the first 18 months or 1.5 million cycles [4]. The total bedding in/wear depth did not exceed 0.41 mm. If creep was the cause of dimension changes there was nothing to suggest that this was a continuous process. **Creep of the UHMWPE cup is of academic interest only; the volumetric changes are primarily due to wear** [4].

References

1. Rose RM, Nusbaum HJ, Schneider H, Ries M, Paul I, Crugnola A, Simon SR, Radin EL. On the true wear rate of ultra-high molecular weight polyethylene in the total hip prosthesis. J Bone Joint Surg (Am). 1980;62A:537–49.
2. Isaac GH, Dowson D, Wroblewski BM. An investigation into the origins of time-dependent variations in penetration rates with Charnley acetabular cups – wear, creep or degradation? Proc Inst Mech Eng. 1996;210:209–16.
3. Hall RM, Unsworth A, Siney P, Wroblewski BM. Wear in retrieved Charnley acetabular sockets. Proc Inst Mech Eng. 1996;210:197–207.
4. Wroblewski BM, Siney PD, Dowson D, Collinson SN. Prospective clinical and joint simulator studies of a new total hip arthroplasty using alumina ceramic heads and cross-linked polyethylene cups. J Bone Joint Surg (Br). 1996;78-B:280–5.

Chapter 34
Factors Affecting Wear of the UHMWPE Cup

It is remarkable that the material, ultra high molecular weight polyethylene (UHMWPE), not specifically formulated for use in the human body, has withstood nearly 50 years under conditions of human activities and function of the hip joint. UHMWPE followed the rapidly wearing PTFE. The possibility of long-term problems resulting from wear, were considered. In the initial reports of this method of treatment the emphasis was primarily on the design of the components, surgical technique, clinical results and the early complications.

In the first publication of the clinical results [1] (1972), wear of the cup was established from examination of annual radiographs. The range of total penetration was from 1 mm in 5 years to no measurable wear in 7 years. The mean penetration rate was 0.13 mm/year. Direct wear measurements were carried out on seven explanted cups.

Increasing follow-up generated revisions and offered an opportunity to study explanted components in detail. It was becoming clear that wear and loosening of the UHMWPE cup was the most likely long-term problem. It was, therefore, essential to study factors affecting wear; the information would be essential for further developments.

Cup Position: Medialised Verses Rim Support?

Medialisation of the cup, by deep reaming of the acetabulum, was Charnley's attempt to reduce wear and loosening of the ultra high molecular weight polyethylene cup in his hip replacement. In a review of 1,344 cases, with a follow-up to 44 years, we compared radiographic loosening of the cup in two groups of patients; those with medialised and rim supported cups.

The medialised cup where: "the socket was placed very deep in the acetabulum" [1] and the rim support cup: where transverse reaming of the acetabulum,

© Springer International Publishing Switzerland 2016   267
B.M. Wroblewski et al., *Charnley Low-Frictional Torque Arthroplasty of the Hip:
Practice and Results*, DOI 10.1007/978-3-319-21320-0_34

preservation of strong bone, and placement of the cup was within the rim of the acetabulum [2].

The details of the two groups of patients are shown in Table 34.1, the reasons for revision in Table 34.2, and the details of patients available for continuing follow-up in Table 34.3.

The cup penetration rates and the radiographic cup loosening, with the follow-up to 44 years, for all hips, are shown in Figs. 34.1 and 34.2.

With the follow-up to about 10 years there was no difference in the wear rates between the two groups, but the group with rim supported cups had a higher incidence of radiographic cup loosening at comparable follow-up and lower total penetration.

With the follow-up past 10 years both groups showed a continuing reduction in wear rates, but it was slightly more marked in the group with medialised cups.

Table 34.1 Patient demographics of the two groups

	Cup position	
	Medialised	Rim support
Number of patients	479	549
Number of LFAs	638	706
Mean age at operation – years (range)	40.5 (17–51)	41.9 (15–50)
Mean weight – kg (range)	62.5 (30–102)	68.2 (32–108)
Mean follow-up – years (range)	17.9 (1–44)	18 (1–40)
Mean cup wear rate – mm/year (range)	0.09 (0.01–0.71)	0.1 (0.01–0.67)
Mean cup wear total – mm (range)	1.48 (0.1–7.5)	1.65 (0.1–8.0)
Lost to follow-up		
Hips (%)	14 (2.2)	28 (4)
Patients (%)	13 (2.7)	25 (4.6)
Deaths		
Hips (%)	121 (19.0)	113 (16.0)
Patients (%)	91 (19.0)	76 (13.8)
Revisions		
Hips (%)	169 (26.5)	161 (22.8)
Patients (%)	137 (28.6)	134 (24.4)

Table 34.2 Indications/findings at revision

	Cup position	
Findings at revision	Medialised	Rim support
Infection – number (%)	11 (1.70)	12 (1.7)
Dislocation	2 (0.31)	5 (0.7)
Loose/worn cup	122 (19.1)	124 (17.6)
Loose stem	51 (8.0)	46 (6.5)
# stem	18 (2.8)	7 (1.0)
Unexplained pain	1 (0.16)	1 (0.14)
Loose cup radiological – number (%)	178 (28.0)	151 (21.4)

Table 34.3 Cup position – patients attending follow-up. No revisions

	Cup position	
	Medialised	Rim support
Number of patients	238	314
Number of LFAs	334	404
Mean age at operation – years (range)	40.8 (20–50)	42.3 (20–50)
Mean follow-up – years (range)	22.6 (10–44)	21.5 (10–40)
Mean cup wear rate – mm/year (range)	0.07 (0.01–0.31)	0.07 (0.01–0.3)
Mean cup wear total – mm (range)	1.48 (0.1–7.5)	1.5 (0.1–8.0)
Loose cup radiological – number (%)	60 (18)	47 (11.6)

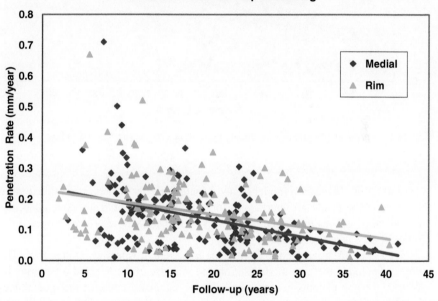

Fig. 34.1 Cup position medialised v rim support. Rate of cup penetration and radiographic cup loosening

The lower incidence of radiographic cup loosening to 10 years and continuing lower wear rate at 10–44 years in the group with medialised cups do support the Charnley concept. However, with the follow-up past 10 years the group with medialised cups had a higher incidence of radiographic cup loosening at comparable follow-up despite the lower total penetration.

Suggestions have often been made that tissue reaction to UHMWPE wear particles is the cause of component loosening [3]. Lower wear rate, lower total penetration and yet a higher incidence of cup loosening in the medialised cup group, while higher wear rate and higher total penetration and yet lower incidence of radiographic cup loosening in the group with rim supported cups does not support such a theory.

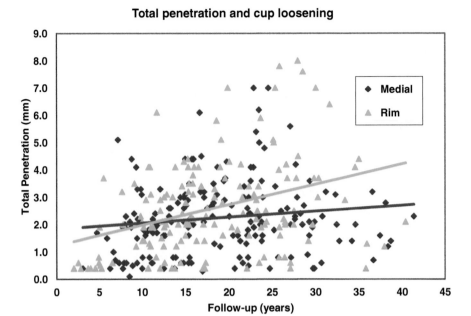

Fig. 34.2 Cup position medialised v rim support. Total cup penetration and radiographic cup loosening

Bonnin et al. [4] used a model to investigate the effect of cup medialisation on the forces at the head-cup interface in total hip replacement. They concluded that "medialisation of the cup decreased stresses at the head-cup interface … even if the global offset was not restored." [4].

Terrier et al. [5] attempted to resolve the issue in a prospective clinical trial. The authors concluded that cup medialisation and increase of the femoral offset may be effective in some patients but must be balanced against the loss of the medial acetabular bone stock. Suggestion that medialisation of the cup results in "additional loss of medial acetabular bone stock" [5] appears to be correct.

In clinical practice preservation of good acetabular bone stock, correct cementing, reduced diameter neck [6] together with a combination of low-wearing materials: alumina ceramic and cross-linked polyethylene [7] is the practical way forward.

Cement Ingress: Its Role in Cup Wear [8]

Fifty nine Charnley acetabular cups, 38 with femoral stems obtained following revision, were examined visually, with CAMSCAN 3/30 BM scanning electron microscope, and Rotary Talysurf 4.

The findings were:

- Majority of the cups (86 %) showed pitting of the articulating area; 49 % had particles of acrylic cement embedded in the surface (Figs. 34.3 and 34.4).
- There was damage to the surface finish of the stainless steel heads increasing the roughness from 0.02 to 0.07 μmRA – an increase in peak – valley difference of 3.5 times (Figs. 34.5, 34.6 and 34.7).
- In 34 % of specimens the outer surface of the cups, which had areas devoid of acrylic cement, showed erosion of the UHMWPE due to its movement against the bony acetabulum (Fig. 34.8).

The conclusions were

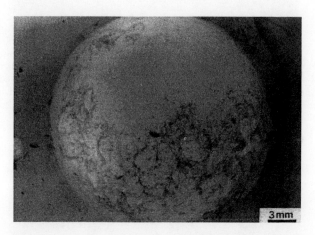

Fig. 34.3 Extensive pitting of the articulating surface of the cup due to cement ingress. [8] Reprinted with permission from Isaac GH, Atkinson JR, Dowson D, Wroblewski BM: The role of cement in the long term performance and premature failures of Charnley low friction arthroplasties. Engineering in Medicine, vol. 15 no. 1 19–22. Copyright © 1986, © SAGE Publications

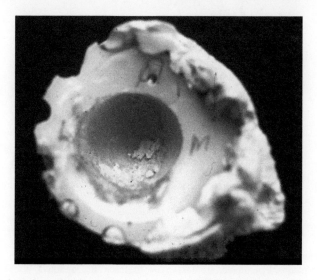

Fig. 34.4 Explanted cup showing extensive pitting of articulation and cement ingress

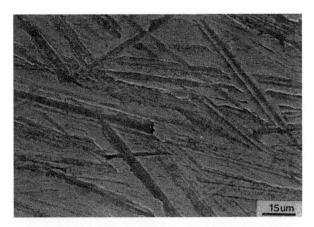

Fig. 34.5 Electron micrograph showing scratches on the surface of explanted femoral component. [8] Reprinted with permission from Isaac GH, Atkinson JR, Dowson D, Wroblewski BM: The role of cement in the long term performance and premature failures of Charnley low friction arthroplasties. Engineering in Medicine, vol. 15 no. 1 19–22. Copyright © 1986, © SAGE Publications

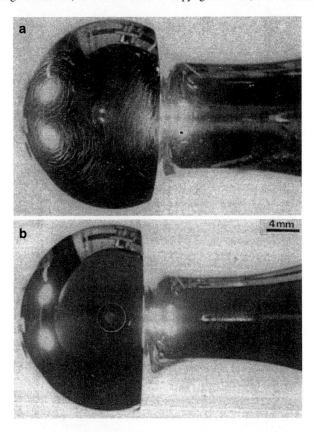

Fig. 34.6 New and explanted metal femoral components showing scratches on explanted component. [8] Reprinted with permission from Isaac GH, Atkinson JR, Dowson D, Wroblewski BM: The role of cement in the long term performance and premature failures of Charnley low friction arthroplasties. Engineering in Medicine, vol. 15 no. 1 19–22. Copyright © 1986, © SAGE Publications

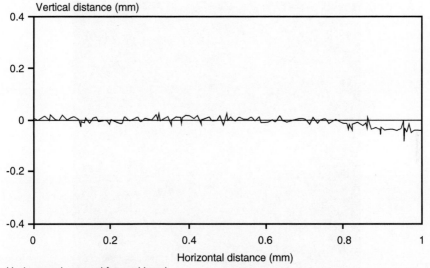

Undamaged, unused femoral head

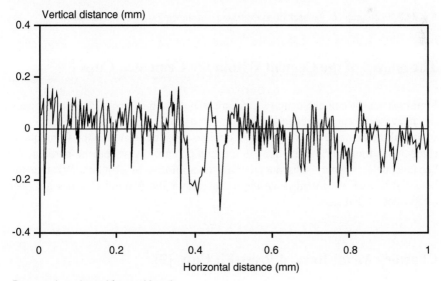

Damaged, explanted femoral head

Fig. 34.7 Surface profile of a new and an explanted femoral component head measured by Rotary Talysurf (Reproduced with permission from Isaac et al. [13])

– Ingress of acrylic cement, with its opacifiers, Barium Sulphate and Zirconium Dioxide, damage the surface finish of the metal head increasing its roughness 3.5 times, on average, and was the likely cause for increasing the rate of cup wear.
– Erosions of the external surface of the cups in the areas devoid of acrylic cement, could only occur <u>after</u> cup loosening; loosening of the cup must precede the external wear.

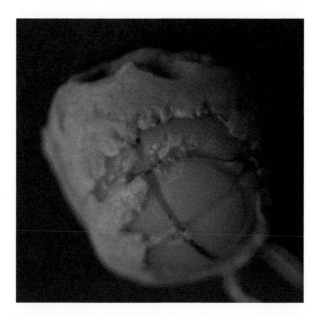

Fig. 34.8 Photograph of the back of an explanted cup showing wear of the plastic

The Source of the Cement Within the Cemented Cups [9]

Ingress of acrylic cement, damage to the metal head of the femoral component causing increased wear, has been demonstrated [8]. It was important to identify the
source of the cement. Clearly the most obvious must be related to the technique of
cement handling during fixation of the components. Any cement particle that
becomes detached may subsequently be drawn into the articulation. Whether this
potential source of cement is on the acetabular or the femoral side has not been
established at that stage.

Charnley Metal-Backed Press-Fit Cups [9]

Fifteen Charnley metal-backed press-fit cups used with cemented stems, were available from post-mortems. The mean follow-up was 10.7 years (6.7–17). No cement
was found in any of the cups but seven showed areas which were consistent with the
cement having been present. The conclusion was that other than particles of cement
being left in the operative field – the source must be mainly the acetabular side.
Improvements in surgical technique and the use of flanged cups was recommended
(Unfortunately the femoral components were not available; they were part of
Charnley's studies of bone-cement interface).

Surface Topography of Explanted Femoral Head [10]

Surface roughness values of 37 explanted and five new Charnley prostheses were examined using Rodenstock RM 600 non-contacting profilometer and scanning electrouniscope.

The conclusions were:-

– Damage to the metal femoral head occurs in vivo. It is localised in form of scratches.
– No overall discernable direction could be observed.
– No correlation was found between the degree of roughness and the follow-up suggesting that the damage occurs **early**, possibly even at surgery.

Undamaged Metal Head: A Feature in the Long-Term Successful Results [11]

The deleterious effects of the increased surface roughness of the head of the femoral component could be anticipated from basic knowledge of factors affecting wear. What has not been shown before was that maintaining a good quality surface finish of the stainless steel head, under clinical conditions, would have the benefit of low wear.

Examination of the heads of four Charnley stems, at an average of 20 years after implantation, has shown an average surface roughness of 0.031 µm (range 0.008–0.102 µm) as compared with 0.019 µm (range 0.008–0.31 µm) for the production stems, and 0.05 µm as recommended by the British Standards Institution and the International Standards Organisation (Fig. 34.9).

– The degree of roughness was greater when measured in the coronal plane suggesting that the main direction of hip movement takes place in the sagittal plane.
– The mean rate of cup penetration was 0.022 mm/year and none of the cups were loose either radiologically or on examination at revision of the stem.
– The information obtained indicated cup fixation can remain secure for up to 20 years, PROVIDED: the surface finish of the stainless steel head is not only achieved but maintained. Under such conditions neither wear nor loosening of the cup was a problem.

Wear Properties of UHMWPE from Explanted Cups [12]

Theoretical consideration indicated that UHMWPE, implanted in the human body, and under repeated sliding load, would be subject to two factors: wear and degradation. Examination of explanted UHMWPE cups would thus offer very useful

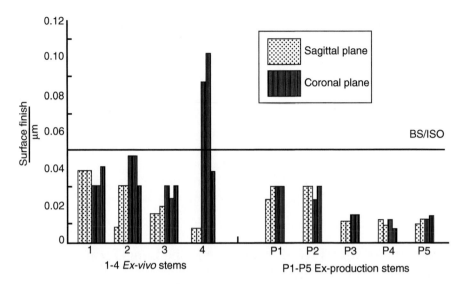

Fig. 34.9 Quality of surface finish of the heads of four Charnley components – compared with five production models (Reproduced with permission from Wroblewski et al. [11])

information and possibly distinguish between the effects of degradation on one hand and wear and degradation on the other.

The study was undertaken by the Imperial College, London. Twelve Charnley UHMWPE acetabular cups, retrieved at revision, were examined. Wear and depth of penetration was measured using acrylic casts and the shadowgraph technique. Wear test specimens were machined from the inner aspect of the cups from the worn sections; to test for the effects of wear and degradation, and from the unworn sections to test for the effects of degradation only.

The findings are summarised:

– The penetration rate of the cups was not related to the wear resistance of the material: wear coefficient was not related to the rate of cup wear whether this was low <0.05 mm/year, medium 0.1–0.2 mm/year or high >0.5 mm/year.
– Large variations in the clinical penetration rates could not be explained by variations in the wear resistance of the explanted material.
– There was no evidence of time dependent degradation in wear resistance of UHMWPE with a follow-up to 17.5 years.

Evidence obtained from the study indicated that there was no obvious variation in the quality of UHMWPE, nor its degradation in the human body over a period of up to 17.5 years, which would account for the variations in the rate of wear as observed in clinical practice.

The findings are very encouraging but further investigation into factors affecting wear is essential.

References

1. Charnley J. Total prosthetic replacement of the hip. Physiotherapy. 1967;53:407–9.
2. Charnley J. Low friction arthroplasty of the hip. Theory and practice. Berlin: Springer; 1979. p. 220–41.
3. Harris WH. The problem is osteolysis. Clin Orthop Relat Res. 1995;31:46–53.
4. Bonnin MP, Archbold PH, Basiglini L, Selmi TA, Beverland DE. Should the acetabular cup be medialised in total hip arthroplasty. Hip Int. 2011;21(4):428–35.
5. Terrier A, Florencio FL, Rudiger HA. Benefit of cup medialisation in total hip arthroplasty is associated with femoral anatomy. Clin Orthop Relat Res. 2014;472:3159–65.
6. Wroblewski BM, Siney PD, Fleming PA. Effect of reduced diameter neck stem on incidence of radiographic cup loosening and revisions in Charnley low-frictional torque arthroplasty. J Arthroplasty. 2009;24:10–4.
7. Wroblewski BM, Siney PD, Fleming PA. Low friction arthroplasty of the hip using alumina ceramic and cross-linked polyethylene. A 17 year follow-up report. J Bone Joint Surg (Br). 2005;87-B:1220–1.
8. Isaac GH, Atkinson JR, Dowson D, Wroblewski BM. The role of cement in the long-term performance and premature failure of Charnley low friction arthroplasties. Eng Med. 1986;15(1):19–22.
9. Isaac GH, Wroblewski BM, Atkinson JR, Dowson D. Source of the cement in the Charnley Hip. J Bone Joint Surg (Br). 1990;72-B:149–50.
10. Hall RM, Unsworth A, Siney PD, Wroblewski BM. The surface topography of retrieved femoral heads. J Mater Sci Mater Med. 1996;7:739–44.
11. Wroblewski BM, McCullagh PJ, Siney PD. Quality of the surface finish of the head of the femoral component and the wear rate of the socket in long-term results of the Charnley low-friction arthroplasty. Proc Inst Mech Eng. 1992;206:181–3.
12. Weightman B, Swanson SAV, Isaac GH, Wroblewski BM. Polyethylene wear from retrieved acetabular cups. J Bone Joint Surg. 1991;73-B:806–10.
13. Issac GH, Wroblewski BM, Atkinson JR, Dowson D. A Tribological study of retrieved hip prostheses. Clin Orthop Relat Res 1992;276:115–125.

Chapter 35
Factors Affecting Wear. Patient Activity Level

… wear is related more to the grade of functional activity than the weight of the subject. (1973).

It was clear that any study of factors affecting wear of the UHMWPE cup had to take patient activity level into account. Although there is agreement as to its importance, translating "activity level" into some standard and uniformly acceptable form has proved more difficult. Other than enumerating some common activities often related to sport or employment, the tendency has often been to present anecdotal, single case successes.

Theoretical Considerations

We set out to assess patients' activity level as expressed in terms of load and sliding distance at the level of articulation.

It was assumed that walking is the main activity and the highest load to which the hip joint is subjected, other than occasionally. If leg length, stride length and the time taken to walk a measured distance were known, then the sliding distance at the level of the articulation could be calculated as a simplified to and fro linear motion.[1]

---

[1] In the study by Feller et al. [1] an assumption was made that the sliding path at the articulation is linear but reciprocating. This is an approximation; the pelvis does not remain level during the walking cycle. Elevation and dipping of the pelvis during the weight-bearing and the swing phase results in sliding in the coronal plane. The resultant sliding pattern is a combination of movement both in the saggital and coronal planes: resembling a figure 8. Hence the true sliding distance at the articulation is greater than calculated from the linear, reciprocating pathway.

© Springer International Publishing Switzerland 2016
B.M. Wroblewski et al., *Charnley Low-Frictional Torque Arthroplasty of the Hip:*
Practice and Results, DOI 10.1007/978-3-319-21320-0_35

Clinical Assessment of Activity Levels [1]

Patients selected for the study fulfilled two set criteria: the follow-up was not less than 8 years and patients considered the outcome a success. Seventy nine patients, 109 Charnley LFAs, were included in the study.

A detailed questionnaire, completed at an interview, was used as an indication of activities over a typical 1 week period. As a result each patient was assigned to a one of five activity grade based on the estimated distance walked during 1 week (The distance walked during 1 week varied from 1 km to more than 25 km). In order to validate the estimates, as recorded in questionnaires, 21 patients were selected for pedometer studies. Their leg and stride length, as well as the time to walk a measured distance, were recorded.

Detailed statistical analysis has shown that:

- For the pedometer study group there was a highly significant correlation between the estimated and the measured distance walked.
- There was inverse, but still significant, correlation between the assigned activity grade and the time to walk the measured distance.
- The mean estimated sliding distance, at the level of the articulation: was 20,638 m/year (20.638 km) with a very wide range of 984–67408 m/year (0.984–67.408 km). It correlated very significantly with the assigned activity grade.
- There was statistically highly significant correlation between the activity grade and the wear of the UHMWPE cup and between the sliding distance per year at the level of the articulation and the wear of the cup.
- There was no statistically significant correlation between gender, underlying hip pathology, patients' age, weight, height, leg or stride length, or the product of weight and the length of follow-up – and cup wear.

Activity of Patients with Total Hip Replacement: Pedometer Study [2, 3]

Previous study [1] established significant correlation between patients activity level, sliding distance at the level of the articulation and the rate of wear of the UHMWPE cup. Studies were extended [2, 3] in order to:

- Compare activity level of patients with total hip replacement and normal subjects.
- Establish the number of loading cycles to which the prosthesis should be subjected in joint simulation studies of implant performance.
- Establish an experimental procedure for the assessment of the role of activity to the measurement of wear rates of the UHMWPE cup.

Two groups of subjects were studied using pedometers.

- 63 patients with Charnley LFA carried out 0.9–26.4 years previously.
- 24 normal subjects.

Most wore pedometers for four consecutive weeks.
The conclusions were:

- Hip replacement did not restrict activity level when compared with normal subjects.
- Patients with hip arthroplasty were generally more active than hitherto considered.
- Young patients, under the age of 44 years, were more active than their normal counterparts.
- The number of loading cycles on each leg, in a 1 year period, decreased with increasing age and was 1.69, 1.53 and 1.37 ($\times 10^6$) for patients aged 40, 50 and 60 respectively.
- The wide scatter of activity level was not unexpected and must be accepted as one of the factors observed in clinical practice where the wide scatter of wear rates has been frequently reported.
- There was a decline in the activity levels of both normal and arthroplasty patients with increasing age.

The mean number of loading cycles per year was in the region of 1,500,000. This has practical implications for any study using simulated activity levels to assess new materials for their possible use in total hip replacement.

References

1. Feller JA, Kay PR, Hodgkinson JP, Wroblewski BM. Activity and socket wear in the Charnley low friction arthroplasty. J Arthroplast. 1994;9(4):341–5.
2. Goldsmith AAJ, Dowson D, Wroblewski BM, Siney PD, Fleming PA, Lane JM, Stone MH, Walker R. Comparative study of the activity of total hip replacement patients and normal subjects. J Arthroplast. 2001;16(5):613–9.
3. Goldsmith AAJ, Dowson D, Wroblewski BM, Siney PD, Fleming PA, Lane JM. The effect of activity levels of total hip arthroplasty patients on socket penetration. J Arthroplast. 2001;16(5):620–7.

Chapter 36
Wear of UHMWPE Cup and Consequences

Charnley was probably the first to suggest that "*late failure ... may be expected from tissue reaction to particles abraded from the bearing surfaces*".

Pain relief is the hallmark of a successful total hip arthroplasty; the natural symptomatic joint is replaced with an artificial, neuropathic spacer functioning within a foreign body bursa.

Activity level achieved after the operation is not a characteristic of a particular design nor the method of component fixation, provided it remains secure when under load, it is a reflection of patient selection for the operation.

This method of surgery demands not only the clinical skill of patient selection but also the practical skill of component fixation. That skill will be tested severely by the repeated loading of the implant within the ever changing skeleton.

The consequences of improved function can be expressed as load and sliding distance at the articulation and quantified as wear.

Wear has two basic elements: wear products shed into the tissues and structural changes of the articulation.

We are concerned here with wear of the UHMWPE cup and its effect on component fixation.

Since absolute rigidity does not exist in nature, the quality of component fixation, in the context of the neuropathic spacer, total hip arthroplasty, cannot be defined in terms that may be acceptable to all. By analogy failure of fixation cannot be defined in terms of clinical results. Hence, clinical results cannot be expected to reflect the mechanical state of the arthroplasty: the quality of component fixation.

The role of UHMWPE wear particles, the tissue reaction they stimulate and the possible effects on component fixation, continues to be of wide interest.

It was Willert and Semlitsch [1] who were quite definite in their conclusions derived from the studies of hip endoprosthesis: cobalt chromium alloy articulating with polyethylene or polyethylene terephthalate. They stated that granulation tissue may act on the neighbouring bone "which is removed by extensive resorption leading to loosening of the prosthesis".

© Springer International Publishing Switzerland 2016

B.M. Wroblewski et al., *Charnley Low-Frictional Torque Arthroplasty of the Hip: Practice and Results*, DOI 10.1007/978-3-319-21320-0_36

With an increasing number of publications the terminology changed: "cement disease" gave way to "cementless disease", "particle disease", "poly disease" and "access disease" as the causes of component loosening we proposed.

Eventually "osteolysis" became and continues to be the term used to define not only the effects of tissue reaction to wear particles, but also the cause of component loosening.

What has happened, almost certainly inadvertently, is that radiographic appearances at the bone-cement interface – were ascribed as being due to a definite pathological process- osteolysis – removal of calcium of bone and was now responsible for component loosening.

It is that leap of reasoning: from tissue reaction to UHMWPE wear particles, a very definite entity, to loosening of components, a very definite mode of failure, without consideration of the mechanical causes of failure, that has resulted in a number of changes in materials, design and methods of component fixation.

Study of alternative materials is essential but must be planned with caution and in the full knowledge of past experience. Comparable follow-up is essential.

Attempts at counteracting tissue response to UHMWPE wear particles is unlikely to be of long term value. It is unlikely that the human body will respond specifically to a particular implant material, provided its chemical state, immunological response or mutation potential has not been affected. To argue otherwise would be to accept the unlimited possibilities of response to the vast ingenuity of the inventor and designer. As for the technique of component fixation: "*Surgeons yearn for an easy hip operation*" finds a response in "cementless" implants which aim to replace the technical skill, a commodity that cannot be sold at a profit, with an implant which becomes a profitable product.

It is essential that the mechanical environment of the foreign body bursa – the total hip arthroplasty – be examined for any possible improvements before attempting wholesale changes based on incomplete evidence.

Wear of UHMWPE Cup: Mechanical Consequences

Nowhere in the locomotor system would liaison with university departments of engineering and colleges of technology be more rewarding than in the biomechanics of the hip joint.

Changes in geometry resulting from wear are easily understood and can be reproduced and tested experimentally. It is here that collaboration with scientific institutions and industry is invaluable.

Charnley commented on this aspect half a century ago: Basic mechanical changes resulting from wear will be discussed briefly – Friction characteristics, frictional torque, decreasing rigidity of the cup wall, impingement, external cup wear and finally the incidence of cup loosening in relation to cup penetration. It must be accepted that the changes are inter-related and all contribute to cup loosening.

Changes in Friction Characteristics

Hall et al. (1994) [2] studied 54 explanted and 5 new Charnley hip prostheses. Frictional resistance was measured using the Durham hip function simulators both under dry and lubricated conditions.

The friction factor for the new prostheses showed normal, bell-shaped scatter. This distribution was skewed for the explanted prostheses; although most retained comparable friction values, a significant number showed increased frictional resistance. Friction factor did not increase with the depth of cup penetration or follow-up. There was no clear correlation between friction factor and whether the cups revised were loose or exchanged for other reasons. The conclusion was that increased friction alone is unlikely to be responsible for the increasing rate of cup loosening observed with increasing depth of cup penetration.

Frictional Torque

The benefits of the low frictional torque have been discussed in Chap. 31.

Decreasing Rigidity of the Cup Wall

Increasing depth of cup penetration reduces the thickness of the cup wall increasing the amplitude of deflection under load. This aspect has not been a subject of detailed studies. Its clinical significance is not easy to establish. Careful examination of serial radiographs may reveal the evidence: fracture of the wire marker in the region of the direction of cup wear with fracture of the acetabular cement, (Fig. 36.1) localised cavitation around cement peg (Fig. 36.2) and wear-out and fracture of the cup without cup loosening (Fig. 36.3) [3].

Impingement

Charnley et al. [4] were the first to suggest that more than 5 mm wear might cause impingement of the neck of the prosthesis against the inner rim of the cup and cause loosening at the bone-cement interface. Pursuing the concept of impingement Hall et al. [5] examined 74 explanted Charnley cups.

– A strong positive association was observed between penetration depth and impingement irrespective of whether the neck diameter was 12.5 mm or 10 mm.
– Reducing the diameter of the neck of the stem from 12.5 to 10 mm reduced the probability of impingement.

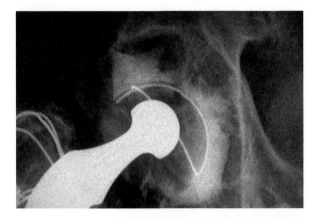

Fig. 36.1 Fracture of the wire marker in the region of the direction of cup wear with fracture of the acetabular cement

Fig. 36.2 Wear of the cup and localised cavitation around cement peg

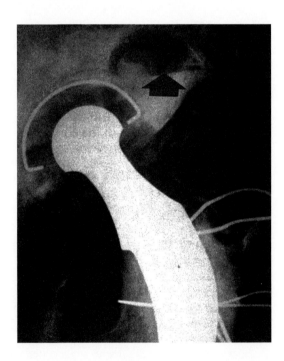

- With the 12.5 mm diameter neck there was 50 % probability of impingement at zero penetration.
- With the 10 mm diameter neck the 50 % probability of impingement did not occur until 2 mm of cup penetration had been reached.
- The conclusion was: **"if impingement is a problem then the reduced diameter neck appears to be a solution in cutting rates of long-term cup loosening"**[5].

Fig. 36.3 Wear and
fracture of the UHMWPE
cup. (Note the cup is not
loose - medially)

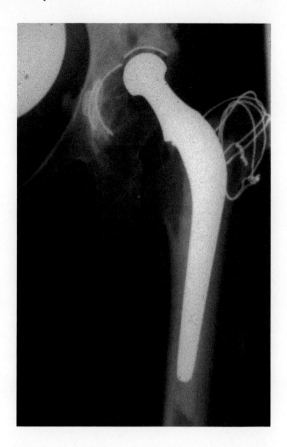

External Cup Wear [6, 7]

Examination of 159 explanted cups showed areas of wear on the outer surface. It
was found in 53 (33 %) of cups. Their size increased with follow-up and depth of
cup wear. Appearances indicate a 'to and fro' rocking movement against the acetabular bone – a mechanical cause.

Depth of Cup Penetration and Incidence of Cup Loosening

Studies on the subject of cup wear (penetration) and loosening are summarised.

Patients under the age of 40 at surgery (1984). Seventy one patients; 104 LFAs,
mean age of 32 years at LFA and a follow-up of 9.3 years (4–17) showed increasing
incidence of cup migration with increasing depth of cup penetration (Table 36.1,
Fig. 36.4) [8].

Table 36.1 Details of 1984 study. Correlation between depth of cup penetration (mm) and the incidence of cup migration (%)

Cup penetration (mm)	0	1	2	3	4	5	6
Number of LFAs	13	37	20	16	11	6	1
Number of cups migrating	0	0	1	2	4	3	1
% of cups migrating	0	0	5.0	12.5	36.0	50.0	100

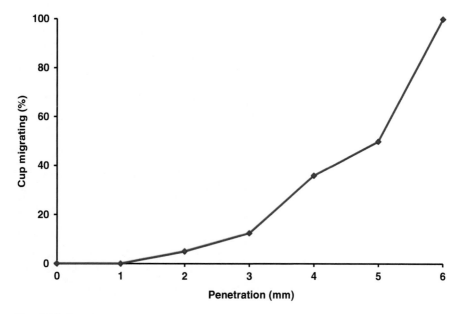

Fig. 36.4 Correlation between depth of cup penetration (mm) and the incidence of cup migration (%)

Fifteen to 21 year results (1986). Ninety three patients, (103 LFAs), mean age of 53 years (20–71) and a mean follow-up of 16.6 years (15–21) (Table 36.2, Fig. 36.5) [9].

Eighteen to 26 year results. (1993). One hundred and eighty five patients, (193 LFAs), mean age of 47 years (28.6–68.1) and a mean follow-up of 20.8 years (18.1–26) (Table 36.3, Fig. 36.6) [10].

Twenty to 30 year results. (1999). Two hundred and sixty one patients, (320 LFAs), mean age of 43 years (17–68) and a mean follow-up of 22 years 10 months (20–30) (Table 36.4, Fig. 36.7) [11].

Follow-up to 33 years. (2002). One thousand and ninety two patients (1434 LFAs), mean age of 41 years (12–57) and a mean follow-up of 15 years 1 month (10–33 years) (Table 36.5, Fig. 36.8) [12].

It is obvious that increasing depth of cup penetration and increasing incidence of cup loosening are very closely related.

Table 36.2 Details of 1986 study. Correlation between depth of cup penetration (mm) and the incidence of cup migration (%)

Cup penetration (mm)	0	1	2	3	4	5	6	7
Number of LFAs	27	28	30	9	4	3	–	2
Number of cups migrating	0	2	5	3	2	2	–	2
% of cups migrating	0	7.1	16.7	33.3	50.0	66.7	–	100

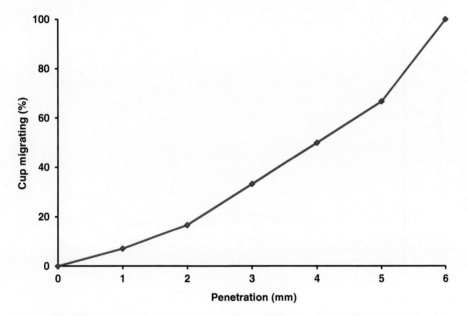

Fig. 36.5 Details of 1986 study. Correlation between depth of cup penetration (mm) and the incidence of cup migration (%)

When total penetration reaches 5 mm the chance of the cup being radiologically loose often exceeds 50 %. Whether revision is undertaken will depend on the regularity of follow-up and the surgeon's awareness of the mechanical problem and not the patient's symptoms.

What is not immediately obvious, but probably even more important, is the fact that with no measurable wear the chances of the cup being loose is less than 2 %. In the collection of publications listed there were 137 cups with no measurable wear. Only two, at a mean follow-up of 16.6 years (15–21), were radiologically loose. This information is very encouraging. If factors affecting wear can be identified and avoided or at least minimised, then the prospects of reducing the incidence of aseptic cup loosening with the Charnley design and technique are very good indeed.

Table 36.3 Details of 1993 Study. Correlation between depth of cup penetration (mm) and the incidence of cup migration (%)

Cup penetration (mm)	0	<=1	<=2	<=3	<=4	<=5	>5
Number of LFAs	10	88	46	32	11	4	2
Number of cups migrating	0	8	8	7	6	3	2
% of cups migrating	0	9	17	22	55	75	100

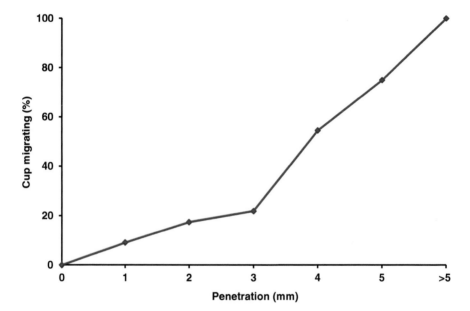

Fig. 36.6 Details of 1993 Study. Correlation between depth of cup penetration (mm) and the incidence of cup migration (%)

The Effect of Cup Inclination

In the description of the surgical technique Charnley advocated a cup inclination, angle open laterally, of 45° and anteversion of not more than 5° to account for the tilt of the pelvis at surgery. The subject of cup position became of interest in the study of long-term results. Because of the complexity, we examined the individual and combined influences of cup inclination and wear on the contact mechanics of the articulation as well as the stress within the cement and bone-cement interface. Experimental findings indicated that contact mechanics at the articulation and cement stress were insensitive to cup inclination of up to 65° and cup penetration of 4 mm [13].

The experimental evidence supports the long-term success of the Charnley concept.

Table 36.4 Details of 1999 Study. Correlation between depth of cup penetration (mm) and the incidence of cup migration (%)

Cup penetration (mm)	0	<=1	<=2	<=3	<=4	<=5	<=6	>6
Number of LFAs	14	121	70	68	28	12	4	3
Number of cups migrating	0	13	11	18	8	4	2	2
% of cups migrating	0	11	16	27	29	33	50	67

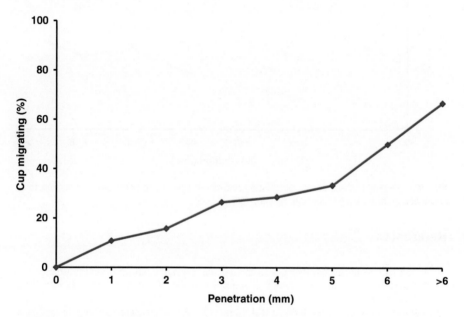

Fig. 36.7 Details of 1999 Study. Correlation between depth of cup penetration (mm) and the incidence of cup migration (%)

Table 36.5 Details of 2002 study: Correlation between depth of cup penetration (mm) and incidence of cup migration (%) and cup revision (%)

Cup penetration (mm)	0	<=1	<=2	<=3	<=4	<=5	<=6	>6
Number of cups	73	754	261	195	91	40	10	10
Number migrating	0	108	76	71	43	24	5	7
% Migrating	0	14	29	36	47	60	50	70
Number revised	0	42	33	36	21	13	3	4
% Revised	0	6	13	18	23	33	30	40

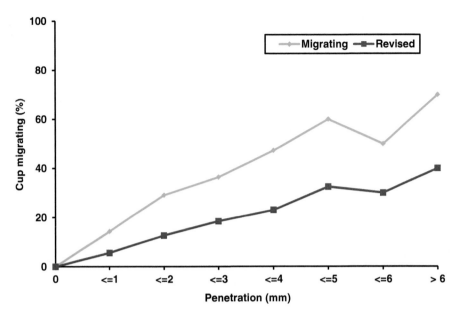

Fig. 36.8 Details of 2002 study: Correlation between depth of cup penetration (mm) and incidence of cup migration (%) and cup revision (%)

References

1. Willert HG, Semlitsch M. Reaction of the articular capsule to artificial joint prostheses. In: Williams D, editor. Biocompatabilty of implant materials. London: Sector Publishing Ltd; 1976. p. 40–8.
2. Hall RM, Unsworth A, Wroblewski BM, Burgess IC. Frictional characterisation of explanted Charnley prostheses. Wear. 1994;175:159–66.
3. Wroblewski BM, Siney PD, Fleming PA. Wear and fracture of the acetabular cup in Charnley low-friction arthroplasty. J Arthroplasty. 1998;13(2):132–7.
4. Charnley J, Halley D. Rate of wear in total hip replacement. Clin Orthop. 1975;112:170.
5. Hall RM, Siney PD, Unsworth A, Wroblewski BM. Prevalence of impingement in explanted Charnley acetabular components. J Orthop Sci. 1998;3:204–8.
6. Wroblewski BM, Lynch M, Atkinson JR, Dowson D, Isaac GH. External wear of the polyethylene socket in cemented total hip arthroplasty. J Bone Joint Surg. 1987;69-B:61–3.
7. Isaac GH, Wroblewski BM, Atkinson JR, Dowson D. Tribological study of retrieved hip prosthesis. Clin Orthop. 1992;278:115–267.
8. Wroblewski BM. Charnley low-friction arthroplasty in patients under the age of 40 years. In: Sevastik Y, Goldie I, editors. The young patient with degenerative hip disease. Stockholm: Almquist & Wiksell; 1984. p. 197–201.
9. Wroblewski BM. 15–21 years results of the Charnley low-friction arthroplasty. Clin Orthop. 1986;211:30–5.
10. Wroblewski BM, Siney PD. Charnley low-friction arthroplasty. Long term results. Clin Orthop. 1993;292:191–201.
11. Wroblewski BM, Fleming PA, Siney PD. Charnley low-frictional torque arthroplasty of the hip. 20 to 30 year results. J Bone Joint Surg (Br). 1999;81-B:427–30.
12. Wroblewski BM, Siney PD, Fleming PA. Charnley low-frictional torque arthroplasty in patients under the age of 51 years. Follow-up to 33 years. J Bone Joint Surg. 2002;84-B:540–3.
13. Hua X, Wroblewski BM, Jin Z, Wang L. The effect of cup inclination and wear on the contact mechanics and cement fixation for ultra high molecular weight polyethylene total hip replacements. Med Eng Phys. 2012;318(3):25–6.

Chapter 37
Wear of the UHMWPE Cup, Tissue Reaction to Wear Particles, Endosteal Cavitation and Component Loosening. Is the Problem Mechanical or Biological?

The failure, if it does eventually supervene, is to be expected from one, or both, of the possible causes: tissue reaction to the particles abraded from the bearing surfaces and mechanical loosening of the bone-cement bond 1967.

As the volume of this material increases it is pumped ... by every movement of the joint and eventually it starts to erode in the plane ... between the plastic cup and the bony bed. 1969.

Charnley introduced ultra high molecular weight polyethylene (UHMWPE) in November 1962 as the material for the cup. It followed the rapidly wearing polytetrafluoroethylene (PTFE, Teflon, Fluon) "The Teflon experience" was neither well documented nor widely known. The information gathered was a caution as to the possibility of future problems with plastic wear particles. The extremely low wear of the UHMWPE was a great encouragement. Although studied in some detail, it was, initially, of radiographic rather than clinical interest. There were no indications of possible problems, certainly not in the short or medium term. There was a more urgent issue to be addressed: the explosion of demand for this type of surgery.

The Willert and Semlitsch Study (1974)

The study of tissue reaction to wear particles generated from metal on plastic articulation was revived by Willert and Semlitsch [1]. They examined 123 explanted endoprostheses of metal, almost exclusively chrome cobalt, and plastic: polyethylene or polyethylene terephthalate articulations. Their conclusion was stated clearly: "We believe that this was responsible for the loosening of endoprostheses with polyester components because an extensive foreign body reaction was found in the narrow spaces close to the prosthesis as well as in the joint cavity.

Our histological findings are supported by clinical and radiographic observations" [1].

It is probably this very detailed report, supported by easy to understand line drawings of wear particle pathways, that revived the issue of tissue reaction to wear

© Springer International Publishing Switzerland 2016
B.M. Wroblewski et al., *Charnley Low-Frictional Torque Arthroplasty of the Hip: Practice and Results*, DOI 10.1007/978-3-319-21320-0_37

particles in general and component loosening in particular. Questions were not asked, and explanations not given, how did wear particles manage to migrate to "marrow spaces close to the prosthesis."?

With an increasing number of publications on the subject the pattern of "cause and effect" became accepted as the inevitable sequence of events. Radiographic appearances of localised endosteal bone erosion gave rise to the term: "osteolysis." With time, demarcation of bone-cement interface of the cup was labelled: "linear osteolysis." It is not clear who was the first to use the term "osteolysis" what is clear is that the term **osteolysis** has become synonymous with tissue reaction to wear particles – initially UHMWPE **and** the cause of component loosening. Harris summarised his views by stating that a number of observations, which appear to be unrelated, "can be drawn together to support this thesis that osteolysis is the dominant problem in total hip arthroplasty" [2].

(It should be pointed out that OSTEOLYSIS is a term defining "dissolution of bone, applied especially to the removal or loss of the calcium of bone." Dorland's Illustrated Medical Dictionary 39th Edition: 2000 p. 1334).

Radiographic appearances of bone erosion and implant demarcation are now labelled as a **process**: loss of calcium, due to tissue reaction to UHMWPE wear particles. Thus, wear of UHMWPE cup, "osteolysis" and component loosening is now taken as a ready-made explanation for failure without the need to question either the method or the skill of component fixation. It also, almost unintentionally, identifies the apparent culprit: – UHMWPE – and eventually all wear particles.

How, why or when do these UHMWPE wear particles enter "the marrow spaces close to the prosthesis?"

Migration of UHMWPE Wear Particles

Wear particles are generated at the articulating surfaces due to their relative motion under load. It is unlikely that macrophages would be attracted to the metal-plastic articulation; wear particles are more likely to follow the pathways generated by fluid movement within what functionally is a foreign body bursa housing a neuropathic spacer. For the particles to reach "marrow spaces close to the prosthesis" [1] a free pathway must be available. Combined with changes in volume and pressure, erosion, cavitation and "osteolysis" will result – with UHMWPE wear particles – as passengers. It is only at this stage that macrophage reaction may become a part of the mechanism leading to bone resorption. Ingress of UHMWPE particles to narrow spaces must precede any macrophage reaction.

A Controversy?

It is essential to appreciate a controversy does not concern facts but the explanation of the facts. It is the explanation of the facts that becomes the reason for action.

The facts are: wear, wear products, tissue reaction to wear products, bone resorption, endosteal cavitation and component loosening. The explanation of the facts attempts to correlate wear – as volume of UHMWPE particles shed into the tissues – and the incidence of component loosening,

For the purpose of the discussion it is assumed that neither the method nor the clinical application of the method of component fixation, is at fault.

Wear and Loosening of the UHMWPE Cup

Wear and loosening of the UHMWPE cup in the Charnley LFA was considered to be the one factor limiting the life of the arthroplasty [3]. This was the conclusion drawn from a review of 104 LFAs in 71 patients under the age of 40 at the time of the operation at a mean follow-up of 9.3 years (range 4–17). The number of publications on the subject confirmed the pattern [4–7].

Increasing depth of cup penetration releases an increasing volume of UHMWPE wear particles into the tissues which is reflected in the increasing incidence of cup loosening. This would suggest a biological cause of cup loosening.

Wear of the UHMWPE Cup and Stem Loosening

The correlation between the depth of cup penetration and the incidence of cup loosening does not hold for the incidence of stem loosening (Table 37.1, Fig. 37.1). The incidence of stem loosening does not follow the pattern observed with the cup.

In order to gather further information we examined the results in two groups of patients where the rate of cup penetration differed by a factor of 10: 0.2 mm/year compared with 0.02 mm/year [8].

Did the tenfold increase of UHMWPE particles have an effect on stem loosening?

The data is presented graphically in Fig. 37.2.

It is clear that if the volume of UHMWPE wear particles shed into the tissues is the cause of cup loosening, it is certainly not the cause for stem loosening.

The pictorial sequence of events described by Willert and Semlitsch [1] does not reach the medullary canal with the Charnley cemented stem.

Reducing Neck Diameter: Putting Off Impingement

The reason for reducing the diameter of the neck of the Charnley stem from 12.5 to 10 mm is based on the evidence which indicated that neck impingement on the cup rim is a likely factor leading to cup loosening [9]. Reducing the diameter of the neck of the stem from 12.5 to 10 mm would have no effect on cup wear: volume of

Table 37.1 Depth of cup wear (penetration) mm, and the incidence of cup and stem revision for loosening. Increasing depth of cup penetration has no effect on the incidence of stem revisions

Cup wear (mm)	<1	<2	<3	<4	>4
Number of LFAs	679	263	208	87	89
Number of cups revised	26	48	54	27	33
% of cups revised	3.8	18.3	26.0	31.0	37.1
Number of stems revised	30	24	20	9	7
% of stems revised	4.4	9.1	9.6	10.3	7.9

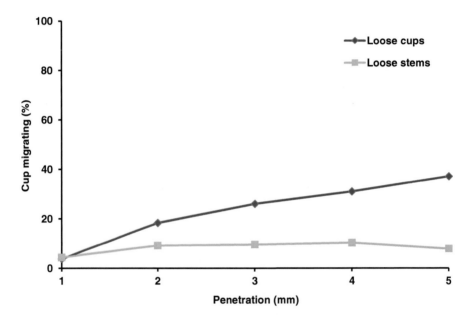

Fig. 37.1 The correlation between the depth of cup penetration and the incidence of component loosening. The incidence of stem loosening does not follow the pattern observed with the cup

UHMWPE particles shed into tissues would be equivalent at comparable depths of cup penetration. However, if impingement of the neck of the stem is the cause of cup loosening, the pattern would remain unchanged, but the incidence of loosening reduced, as predicted by the experimental model [9].

Reduction of the neck diameter from 12.5 to 10 mm was made possible by the introduction of high nitrogen cold formed stainless steel (ORTRON – DePuy International, Leeds, UK.) for the stem manufacture. The new design was fatigue tested and proved at least as strong as the 12.5 mm diameter neck in EN58J and that never failed in clinical practice. It was introduced into clinical practice in October 1983.

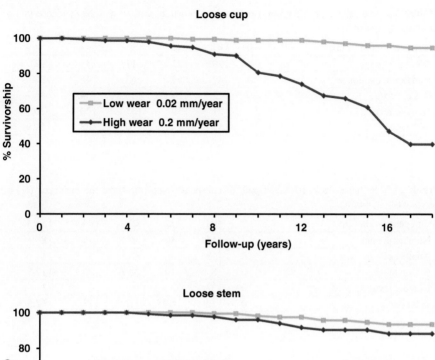

Fig. 37.2 The effect of wear of the UHMWPE cup in the Charnley LFA on the survivorship of the cup and stem

Comparison of the incidence of aseptic cup loosening and revisions, with the two stem designs at comparable depths of cup penetration, with a follow-up over 20 years, has been published [9].

The difference was equivalent to an extra 2 mm of UHMWPE cup penetration – equivalent to 20 years – at 0.1 mm/year – the accepted mean of cup penetration rate. **With the reduced, 10 mm, diameter neck of the Charnley stem, the incidence of cup loosening, at comparable depths of cup penetration, was reduced by 54 %** (Tables 37.2 and 37.3; Figs. 37.3 and 37.4).

Table 37.2 Standard neck. 12.5 mm. Depth of cup penetration (mm) and the incidence (%) of aseptic cup loosening

Cup penetration (mm)	0	<1	<2	<3	<4	>= 4
Number of cups	34	391	222	173	85	67
Number of cup loose	0	47	54	63	46	38
% Cup loose	0	12	24.3	36.4	54.1	56.7
Number revised	0	21	30	35	20	20
% Revised	0	5.4	13.5	20.2	23.5	29.9

Table 37.3 Reduced neck. 10 mm. Depth of cup penetration (mm) and the incidence (%) of aseptic cup loosening

Cup penetration (mm)	0	<1	<2	<3	<4	>= 4
Number of cups	11	161	30	36	15	8
Number of cup loose	0	13	3	8	4	1
% Cup loose	0	8.1	10	22.2	26.7	12.5
Number revised	0	3	2	4	2	1
% Revised	0	1.9	6.7	11.1	13.3	12.5

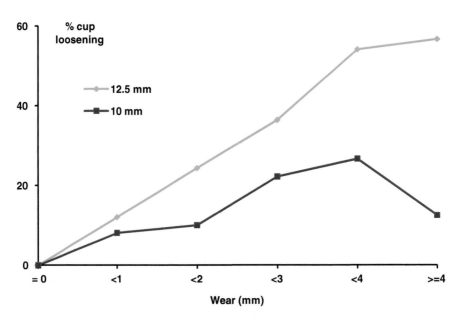

Fig. 37.3 Comparison of standard femoral neck diameter and reduced neck diameter on radiographic cup loosening

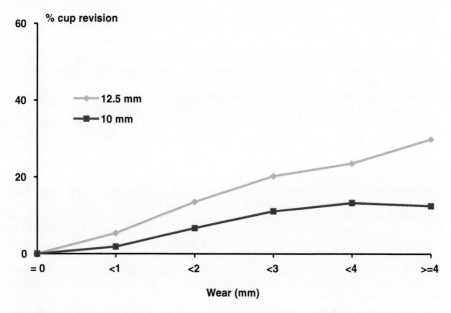

Fig. 37.4 Comparison of standard femoral neck diameter and reduced neck diameter on revision for cup loosening

Intrapelvic PTFE Granuloma

Before concluding this chapter it may be of interest to digress and move some 25 years back.

Examination of radiographs of 160 cases where cemented stem, with a PTFE cup used directly against bone, had shown 53 (33 %) with calcification of intrapelvic granuloma, noted by Charnley. Its appearance was, on average 4.5 years after the original operation. In 40 (25 %) it followed revision to cemented UHMWPE cup. Histology of one such granuloma showed calcification and new bone formation in presence of large numbers of PTFE wear particles. The histology slides were examined by no lesser authority than Professor Willert – Gottingen. His opinion was unambiguous: **Calcification and new bone formation is the evidence of a healing process.** Clearly tissue reaction to PTFE wear particles could <u>not</u> have been per se, the cause of bone destruction [10].

Sequence of events is more in keeping with the problem being mechanical – progressive restriction of the range of movement as well as changes in volume and pressure. This would explain Charnley's comment: "*this material became sealed off … and calcified …*" 1969. Natural healing process.

References

1. Willert HG, Semlitsch M. Reaction of the articular capsule to artificial joint prostheses. In: Williams D, editor. Biocompatabilty of implant materials. London: Sector Publishing Ltd; 1976. p. 40–8.
2. Harris WH. The problem is osteolysis. Clin Orthop. 1995;311:46–53.
3. Charnley J. Total prosthetic replacement of the hip. Physiotherapy. 1967;53:407–9.
4. Wroblewski BM. Charnley low-friction arthroplasty in patients under the age of 40 years. In: Sevastik Y, Goldie I, editors. The young patient with degenerative hip disease. Stockholm: Almquist & Wiksell; 1984. p. 197–201.
5. Wroblewski BM. Direction and rate of socket wear in Charnley low-friction arthroplasty. J Bone Joint Surg (Br). 1985;67-B:757–61.
6. Wroblewski BM, Fleming PA, Siney PD. Charnley low-frictional torque arthroplasty of the hip. 20 to 30 year results. J Bone Joint Surg (Br). 1999;81-B:427–30.
7. Wroblewski BM, Siney PD, Fleming PA. Charnley low-frictional torque arthroplasty in patients under the age of 51 years. Follow-up to 33 years. J Bone Joint Surg. 2002;84-B:540–3.
8. Wroblewski BM, Siney PD, Fleming PA. Wear of the cup in the Charnley LFA in the young patient. J Bone Joint Surg (Br). 2004;86(4):498–503.
9. Wroblewski BM, Siney PD, Fleming PA. Effect of reduced diameter neck stem on incidence of radiographic cup loosening and revisions in Charnley low-frictional torque arthroplasty. J Arthroplasty. 2009;24:10–4.
10. Raut VV, Siney PD, Wroblewski BM, Evans AR. An intrapelvic polytetrafluoroethylene granuloma. Orthop Int. 1995;5:439–44.

Chapter 38
Improving Design and Surgical Technique Reducing the Incidence of Component Loosening

If it be accepted that tissue reaction to UHMWPE particles is the cause of "osteolysis" and component loosening, then it would seem logical to imply that neither improvement in component design nor their fixation would have an effect on the incidence of component loosening.

This reasoning would exonerate the surgeon and the surgical technique, but would certainly condemn the articulating material – the UHMWPE. The natural sequence would be either to alter the tissue response – an unlikely route – or change the materials – as with metal on metal resurfacing. What evidence is there to indicate that both design and the technique play an important role in the incidence of component loosening?

The Cup

The mechanical advantage of the Charnley cup design – flanged or unflanged and pressurisation of the cement, before cup insertion, was tested experimentally. "The ogee-flanged socket gave a consistently high injection pressure which could be maintained throughout the process of polymerization" [1]. The results show clearly the importance of the details of the design, surgical technique and the properties of the cement. They are the important aspects of this type of surgery and must be understood and put into practice at each and every operation. The benefits will be available – long-term.

The Stem

The importance of the stem design [2] attention to the details of the surgical technique [3, 4] and need for follow-up extending past 11 years have been well documented [5]. The benefits are long-term hence the importance of follow-up cannot be overstated. Study of the original publications is recommended.

© Springer International Publishing Switzerland 2016   301
B.M. Wroblewski et al., *Charnley Low-Frictional Torque Arthroplasty of the Hip:
Practice and Results*, DOI 10.1007/978-3-319-21320-0_38

Total Hip Arthroplasty: A Foreign Body Bursa

Total hip arthroplasty, or in fact any total joint arthroplasty is, functionally, a foreign body bursa housing a neuropathic spacer – hence freedom from pain. Bursal fluid will follow the pathways dictated by changes in volume and pressure carrying wear particles and any other debris with it into spaces that may be accessible. If under any mechanical condition a one-way non-return valve condition prevails, local bone erosion will occur. When sufficient endosteal bone is resorbed, as compared with the overlying cortex, cavitation will be seen on radiographs. Their shape will be dictated by the hard materials i.e. cement, metal, and the softer cancellous and cortical bone. The appearance will be that of a compressed ellipsoid defect which will contain UHMWPE or any other debris. This sequence of events is more likely to be present on the femoral side where a one way none-return valve is more like the "piston – cylinder" arrangement of the medullary canal and the implant.

On the acetabular side the same mechanism is less likely to occur, unless around individual cement pegs. Hence the cup is more likely to show a widening gap rather than localised bubble-like cavitation.

Total Hip Replacement: Patterns of Load Transfer

Skeletal changes follow Wolff's Law: Bone responds to function to maintain its strain properties within certain limits. Increasing function will increase bone stiffness while decreasing function will reduce it. The least strained bone will be resorbed. Successful arthroplasty alters the patterns of load transfer.

The Femur

On the femoral side the intramedullary stem invites distal load transfer with resultant strain shielding of the proximal femur and increasing amplitude elastic stem deflection under load. Bursal fluid and its contents will be carried progressively distally. Added to this must be any defects, either as a result of surgical technique, or occurring under function, which may allow bursal fluid ingress.

The Acetabulum

Deflection and deformation of the UHMWPE cup will increase with the depth of cup penetration allowing ingress of bursal fluid and its contents to the bone-implant interface. Impingement of the neck of the stem on the rim of the cup and sheer generated at the bone-implant interface, would act by the same mechanism. Linear rather than cavitatory changes would be the result.

To call this "linear osteolysis" is surely an attempt to force the cause into the "tissue response" theory rather than accept what clearly is a mechanical problem.

One further factor must be taken into consideration. Embroyologically the pelvis has its origin as a membranous bone. Membranous bone, unlike tubular bone, does not readily respond to trauma by callus formation – fibrous tissue is the common response. Why should this be different following the trauma of hip replacement?

The conclusion must be:- bursal fluid and its contents must have access to the bone-implant interface – before any changes can take place. The presence of UHMWPE wear particles may enhance the changes but it is not the primary cause of the changes or component loosening. Presence at the scene of a crime may arouse suspicion but it is not a proof of guilt!

References

1. Shelley P, Wroblewski BM. Socket design and cement pressurisation in the Charnley low-friction arthroplasty. J Bone Joint Surg (Br). 1988;70-B:358–63.
2. Wroblewski BM, Siney PD, Fleming PA. Triple tapered polished cemented stem in total hip arthroplasty. J Arthroplast. 2001;16(8 Suppl):37–41.
3. Wroblewski BM, van der Rijt A. Intramedullary cancellous bone block to improve femoral stem fixation in Charnley low-friction arthroplasty. J Bone Joint Surg (Br). 1984;66-B:639–44.
4. Wroblewski BM, Siney PD, Fleming PA, Bobak P. The calcar femorale in cemented stem fixation in total hip arthroplasty. J Bone Joint Surg (Br). 2000;82-B:842–5.
5. Wroblewski BM, Fleming PA, Hall RM, Siney PD. Stem fixation in the Charnley low-friction arthroplasty in young patients using an intramedullary bone block. J Bone Joint Surg (Br). 1998;80-B:273–8.

Chapter 39
Wear of the Cup. 22.225 mm Alumina Ceramic Head, Charnley Femoral Component and Cross-Linked Polyethylene Cup

Studies of long term results of the Charnley LFA have repeatedly shown increasing incidence of cup migration with an increasing depth of cup penetration.

Factors affecting wear have been studied extensively and it was suggested that ceramics have a potential advantage over metal because of their geometric form and surface topography, together with enhanced hardness and scratch resistance.

A prospective clinical study was initiated in 1986 with 17 patients having 19 LFAs with a 22.225 mm alumina ceramic head on a Charnley femoral stem and a cross-linked polyethylene cup [1] (Fig. 39.1).

Their mean age at surgery was 53.2 years (range, 27–80). The cups were made of a chemically cross-linked polyethylene manufactured using injection moulding in order to reduce cost and wastage of the material.

At the first review [1] in 1996 there had been no revisions but four patients had died and one patient confined to a wheelchair was not fit to attend follow-up. After the initial bedding in to 0.2–0.41 mm total penetration in the first 3 years, there was no further penetration with a follow-up to 8 years. Radiographic wear measurements corresponded with independent laboratory experimental studies [1].

In 1999, 14 hips had been followed-up for over 10 years with none showing further cup penetration [2]. A comparison of three of the patients with bilateral LFAs and stainless steel on ultra high molecular weight polyethylene (UHMWPE) on the contralateral side showed a total penetration of 10–15 times higher using stainless steel (Fig. 39.2).

In the 17 year follow-up report [3] the 11 remaining hips showed no further wear. None of the components were radiologically loose and there was no radiographic appearance of osteolysis.

The latest follow-up of this group was in 2014. From the original group, seven patients had died from unrelated causes and one hip had been revised for deep haematogenous infection at 17 years after the primary operation. In the remaining 11 patients, the mean age at surgery was 46 years (range 26–58) and the mean follow-up was 27.5 years (26–28). After the initial bedding in, none of the hips showed

© Springer International Publishing Switzerland 2016
B.M. Wroblewski et al., *Charnley Low-Frictional Torque Arthroplasty of the Hip: Practice and Results*, DOI 10.1007/978-3-319-21320-0_39

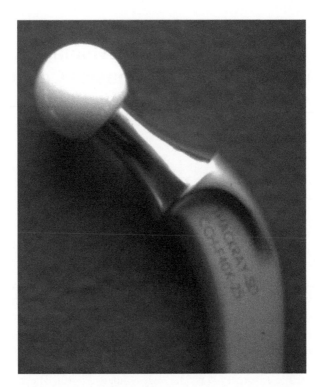

Fig. 39.1 Assembled prosthesis showing an alumina ceramic femoral head on a Charnley femoral component. 1986. The neck of the femoral component having a parallel section and an interposed polyethylene sleeve between the neck and the ceramic head

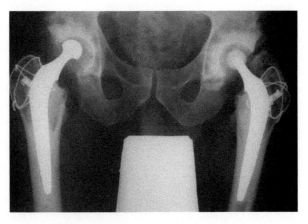

Fig. 39.2 Radiograph showing Alumina ceramic and cross-linked polyethylene articulation on left side and metal on high density polyethylene articulation on right side

further cup penetration and the mean penetration rate was reduced from 0.02 to 0.014 mm/year.

The next stage of study must be the observation of the skeletal changes over the years of normal function in the presence of an unchanging LFA.

References

1. Wroblewski BM, Siney PD, Dowson D, Collins SN. Prospective clinical and joint simulator studies of a new total hip arthroplasty using alumina ceramic heads and cross-linked polyethylene cups. J Bone Joint Surg (Br). 1996;78-B:280–5.
2. Wroblewski BM, Siney PD, Fleming PA. Low-friction arthroplasty of the hip using alumina ceramic and cross-linked polyethylene. A ten year follow-up report. J Bone Joint Surg (Br). 1999;81-B:54–5.
3. Wroblewski BM, Siney PD, Fleming PA. Low-friction arthroplasty of the hip using alumina ceramic and cross-linked polyethylene. A 17-year follow-up report. J Bone Joint Surg (Br). 2005;87-B:1220–1.

Part VII
Follow-Up

Chapter 40
Clinical Results

November 1962 marked the beginning of the era of a new speciality within ortho-paedics – total hip replacement surgery.

This was the date when Charnley working in Wrightington Hospital introduced his method, which has become not only the basis for other designs, but also the source of information for joint replacement in general.

Successful clinical results uncovered the demand for the operation, extended the indications and increased patients' expectations. Assessment before and after surgery using d'Aubigne and Postel's scoring system [1, 2] have demonstrated that the clinical results remain successful [3–6]. At the latest review of our clinical database, 89.7 % of patients are pain free and a further 8.6 % have no more than an occasional discomfort. 74.3 % of patients have normal or near normal function for age, gender and underlying pathology and 77.4 % of patients have full or nearly full range of movement on their operated hip. The mean pre-operative and post-operative clinical scores are shown in Fig. 40.1.

In order to understand the reasons for the clinical success, the need for regular follow-up with good quality radiographs and early intervention in cases of impending failures, it is essential to understand and accept the very simple fact: the arthroplasty is a foreign body bursa housing a neuropathic spacer.

Freedom from pain can be taken for granted subject to correct patient selection and sound fixation of components. It is this aspect of clinical practice that was the driving force that made Charnley persevere with his efforts. Two aspects are worth remembering: first pain at rest, especially at night soon demoralises an individual and becomes almost an absolute indication for surgery, and second memory for pain is very poor.

Study and recording of patients' function is a very complex issue. There is no single method to take all aspects into account and even a most simple parameter will have a vast range. (Olympic games is a perfect example: single event but only one winner.)

© Springer International Publishing Switzerland 2016
B.M. Wroblewski et al., *Charnley Low-Frictional Torque Arthroplasty of the Hip: Practice and Results*, DOI 10.1007/978-3-319-21320-0_40

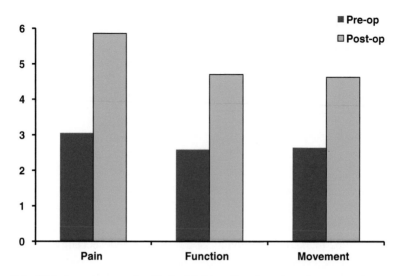

Fig. 40.1 Clinical assessment using Merle d'Aubigne Postel scoring of pre- operative and post-operative pain, function and movement

Anecdotal, single case successes attract attention and increase expectations in prospective patients. Single case spectacular results are not a feature of a particular type of arthroplasty: they are a reflection of patient selection. Patients with multiple disabilities never feature as anecdotal single case successes.

Range of movement of a total hip has been a subject of frequent comments often in context of post-operative dislocation. A "socially acceptable" range is probably adequate for most activities. Excessive range plus the neuropathic nature of the joint invites dislocation.

The Charnley hip replacement, the low frictional torque arthroplasty did not stand still. Improvements, at every level, were brought in purposely as a result of the study of long-term outcomes, findings at re-operations and examination of explanted components.

With increasing demand for THA the emphasis is focused on long-term results. Such studies will invariably identify young patients yet without the benefit of the latest advances in the design, materials or surgical technique.

There is little doubt that the operation of hip replacement will remain a permanent method of treatment for the symptomatic destroyed hip. It could be argued that the success of the operation has delayed if not eliminated altogether the desire for the investigation and treatment of underlying hip pathology in some conditions.

Hip replacement in general and revision surgery in particular has become a sub-speciality within orthopaedics. The demand is not merely for numbers but for the quality, research and development.

The name Charnley remains closely linked with the prosthesis, what is often forgotten is the concept and the technique.

References

1. d'Aubigne MR, Postel M. Functional results of hip arthroplasty with acrylic prosthesis. J Bone Joint Surg (Am). 1954;36-A:451–75.
2. Charnley J. The long-term results of low-friction arthroplasty of the hip as primary intervention. J Bone Joint Surg. 1972;54-B:61–76.
3. Wroblewski BM. 15–21 years results of the Charnley low-friction arthroplasty. Clin Orthop. 1986;211:30–5.
4. Wroblewski BM, Siney PD. Charnley low-friction arthroplasty. Long term results. Clin Orthop. 1993;292:191–201.
5. Wroblewski BM, Fleming PA, Siney PD. Charnley low-frictional torque arthroplasty of the hip. 20 to 30 year results. J Bone Joint Surg (Br). 1999;81-B:427–30.
6. Wroblewski BM, Siney PD, Fleming PA. Charnley low-frictional torque arthroplasty in patients under the age of 51 years. Follow-up to 33 years. J Bone Joint Surg. 2002;84-B:540.

Chapter 41
The Reasons for Follow-Up

I regard it as mandatory that any surgeon aiming to take up the "total prosthesis" should make available to the public a service which can cope with the "maintenance operations." 1966

An important aspect of the use of total prosthetic replacement … is acceptance by the patient of a planned policy of revisions, with the establishment of a centre which holds itself permanently responsible for maintenance operations for this type of surgery. 1966

To countenance the insertion of a total hip replacement into a patient of 25 years of age … without a service station planned and organised … is like selling motor cars without providing mechanics and workshops 1971.

Clinical success of total hip arthroplasty has uncovered the demand in an ageing population, extended the indication for the operation and fuelled by anecdotal single case successes, increased patients' expectations. The operation has almost become a "unit of currency" and a measure of performance of the health services. Increasing demand has put pressure to reduce both the waiting time for the operation and the length of inpatient stay. Combined with the immediate success offered by pain relief, it has, at times, created a false sense of security and a call to abandon follow-up and delay revisions until failures become symptomatic. ("… if it did not trouble the patient it could not be a problem for the surgeon") [1].

Intellectual and technical challenges of ever more complex revisions has resulted in a failure to appreciate that a revision is only an interruption of a process and not some clearly defined advantageous end point. The timing of that intervention must be balanced against problems caused by the delay. The dilemma of the decision to operate for radiographic changes alone, need not present itself if both the patient and the surgeon are aware of the consequences, before the primary operation. **This must be considered as part of informed consent**.

The ultimate value of revision, other than for the individual patient, must be in the information gathered for the benefit of the patients in need of the primary procedures; for that is the real meaning of experience.

© Springer International Publishing Switzerland 2016
B.M. Wroblewski et al., *Charnley Low-Frictional Torque Arthroplasty of the Hip:*
Practice and Results, DOI 10.1007/978-3-319-21320-0_41

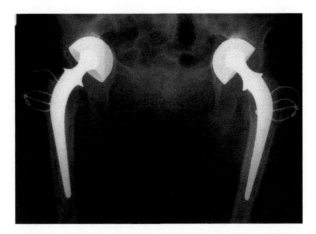

Fig. 41.1 Bilateral Charnley press-fit cups with cemented stems: post operative and follow-up radiograph at 42 years

Establishing a joint "registry" without clearly defined objectives, may encourage a false assumption that because of the volume of information, failures, will at some stage, present themselves identifying the patient, the surgeon, the implant, as well as the cause and mode of failure. Centrally held information absolves the surgeon from reviewing own results. "Guidelines" concerning "performance of prosthesis" or "technique" may discourage attempts at evidence-based innovations. In this context the undefined statement: "there is no such thing as a small change" is an example.

It must be accepted that quality of information does not necessarily increase proportionally with the volume; communal wisdom does not come from individual ignorance.

In order to appreciate the need for regular follow-up and operative intervention for radiographic changes alone, three aspects of this type of surgery must be understood and accepted.

1. The hallmark of success is the immediate pain relief in a correctly selected patient. The reason is simple: the natural, symptomatic joint is replaced with a neuropathic spacer functioning within a foreign body bursa. This fact remains equally valid during the follow-up.
2. Clinical results do not reflect the mechanical state of the arthroplasty. If the natural, symptomatic articulation is replaced with an artificial one, then clearly the articulation cannot be expected to become symptomatic, at any stage. A failing THA will only become symptomatic when the failure of the implant involves living, sensitive tissues e.g. bone. Other than early failures due to infection or obvious dislocation, reliance must be placed on radiographic appearances. It has been adequately documented that radiologically loose components are not necessarily symptomatic [2]. Continuity of the observer method is essential, as is the availability of good quality sequential radiographs.

There is sufficient evidence to indicate that the acetabular side, the cup, is less likely to be symptomatic. Any changes in cup position, does not generate pressure changes within the living bone. An area under compression will almost invariably be mirrored by a space vacated by the movement of the cup. The longest successful results of the Charnley press-fit cup – are just that – press-fit, polished metal-backed cups with UHMWPE inserts and cemented stem (Fig. 41.1).

The femoral side is more likely to be symptomatic. Pressure and volume changes within the medullary canal is the mechanism where the "one-way-non-return valve" comes into play. Even under these circumstances radiographic changes within the medullary canal remain unnoticed "covered" by the cortex. It is for those reasons that changes found at revision are more extensive than anticipated from radiographs.

3. Patient's activity level, after a successful operation, is not a feature of a particular type of arthroplasty; it is a reflection of patient selection. Patients with multiple joint involvement never feature as anecdotal, single case successes. Patients must not expect, and surgeons must not encourage or promise, an unreasonable level of activity after the operation. Relief of pain has a liberating effect which is reflected, amongst others, in physical activity. That level is reached by the patient and is not, nor should it be regarded as an integral part of the operation, and certainly not a part of an "informed consent".

Planned follow-up and revisions, after this type of surgery, must be the accepted practice and must be part of the informed consent for the operation. The frequency must be rationalised in the full knowledge and clear understanding of the underlying principles of the particular design, surgical technique, materials, as well as the results – preferably in terms of patterns of failure and not just the successes.

In Summary

The reasons for follow-up are:

- To establish the patterns of failure.
- To intervene early in cases of impending failures if serious complications, loss of bone stock and ever more complex revisions and poorer outcome are to be avoided.
- To gather the information: clinical, radiographic and that obtained from the examination of the explanted materials, in order to introduce evidence-based improvements.
- To fulfil the clinical, moral and legal obligations of after care.

Experience is not what happens to us – experience is what we do with what happens to us.

References

1. Ring P. Discussion. J Bone Joint Surg (Br). 1973;53B:200.
2. Wroblewski BM, Fleming PA, Siney PD. Charnley low-frictional torque arthroplasty of the hip. 20–30 year results. J Bone Joint Surg (Br). 1999;81-B:427–30.

Chapter 42
Patterns of Failure and Revisions: Guidelines for Follow-Up

Consistency of materials, design and the surgical technique of the Charnley LFA and the long term follow-up results offer detailed information which can be used to set practical guidelines for follow-up.

The clinical results have been recorded since the beginning of the operation in November 1962 up to the end of December 2014, where 25,753 primary LFAs had been carried out. Over this 52 year period, 1,433 (5.6 %) hips had been revised. Survivorship analysis [1] to 37 years where a minimum of 40 hips [2] were still attending was calculated.

The Reason for and the Frequency of Follow-Up

The reasons for follow-up with serial radiographs is to identify problems early and offer revision surgery before complex mechanical failures present clinically. A balance must be struck between the frequency of visits and the value of information obtained. It is in this context that the knowledge of patterns of failure, both by the specific mode and the particular design and technique, is essential. An immediate post-operative radiograph (a-p and lateral) is mandatory. A record, at 1 year after the operation, is an invaluable baseline for comparisons. No specific time intervals can be recommended and "tailoring" the pattern for individual patients becomes the practice. This should be based on the knowledge of underlying pathology, radiographic appearances and progress within the first year after surgery, patient's activity level and the rate of wear of the UHMWPE cup. It is for these reasons that continuity of observer method is essential. Intervals longer than 2 years proved unsatisfactory. Logistics of planning more than 2 years ahead were administratively too complex and non-attendance levels too high and thus a waste of resources with the increasing access to the internet a timely reminder to attend follow-up may be of help. Free access, at short notice, however, must always be available.

© Springer International Publishing Switzerland 2016
B.M. Wroblewski et al., *Charnley Low-Frictional Torque Arthroplasty of the Hip: Practice and Results*, DOI 10.1007/978-3-319-21320-0_42

Anticipating Problems

Pain relief, after total hip arthroplasty, is so spectacular that if the patient's symptoms have not been relieved three possibilities must be considered:

- Complications of surgery.
- Incorrect identification of the original pathology
- Inappropriate patient selection

Complications at Surgery

Attention must be focused on identifying or excluding complications. It is in this context that the availability of good quality sequential radiographs is essential.

Deep Infection

Patients at risk for deep infection include those with previous hip operations, diabetics, patients with rheumatoid arthritis, psoriasis. History of post-surgery urinary tract infection, catheterisation – and in the male – prostatectomy.

Post-operative pain and delayed wound healing is the most sinister combination.

Radiologically – trochanteric separation, wedge erosion of the bone-cement junction at the medial femoral neck, early progressive demarcation of the cup, periostitis at the level of the stem tip and endosteal cavitation at the same level. With any of these, either singly or in combination, infection must be considered until proved otherwise (Fig. 42.1).

Clinical experience indicates that a diagnosis of deep infection is usually suspected, even if not established, within 1 year in the majority of cases with 80.6 % of deep infections having been revised by the eighth year post-op (Fig. 42.2). It is this group of patients that demands regular review – with radiographs and relevant blood tests – every 3 months at least. Although given time infection will declare itself, a high index of suspicion must remain if progress after surgery is slow or symptoms persist. Survivorship at 37 years follow-up was 92.56 % (Fig. 42.2).

Dislocation

The period at risk is days or weeks after surgery. The complication is usually "self-reporting" if associated with pain and loss of mobility and always if manipulation was required after confirming the diagnosis by a radiograph. Episodes of subluxation, or even dislocation, with spontaneous relocation, may be missed. It is for those reasons that this complication remains under-reported. Detailed history of the activity leading to the problem is very helpful. Soft tissue trauma due to tearing of

Fig. 42.1 Radiograph of
an infected LFA

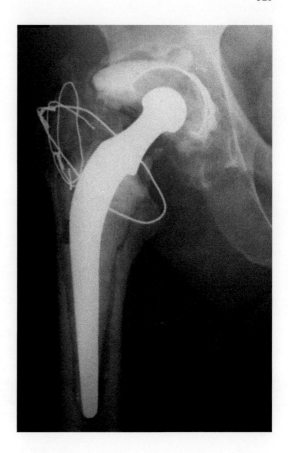

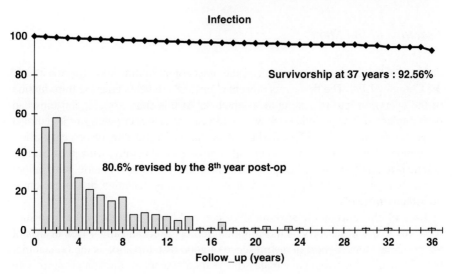

Fig. 42.2 Revision for infection. Incidence and survivorship analysis

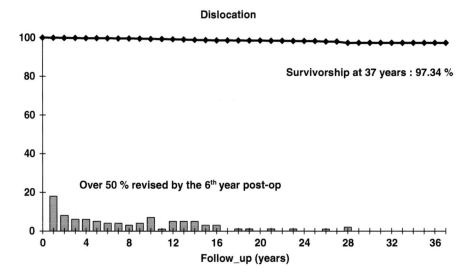

Fig. 42.3   Revision for dislocation. Incidence and survivorship

the capsule by the subluxed, dislocated head, results in pain which may persist for days or even weeks. Review within 6 weeks or so is recommended to either confirm the diagnosis, establish recurrent dislocation as the problem or exclude the more sinister diagnosis – deep infection. Over half of the revisions for dislocation were within 6 years of surgery with revision after the eighth year rare, and often the consequence of wear and resultant cup loosening. The survivorship at 37 years follow-up was 97.34 % (Fig. 42.3).

Fracture of the Stem

Fracture of the stem, was at one stage, the most common indication for revision of the Charnley LFA. The first cases presented in 1968 – 6 years after the introduction of the operation into routine clinical practice. At this stage some 2,500 hips had been implanted. The period at risk was 4–13 years after surgery with survivorship at 37 years – 93.33 % (Fig. 42.4). Radiographic "at risk" signs may be present earlier: separation of the stem from the cement – proximally-laterally, with poor cement mantle proximally-medially. Slip of the stem within the cement mantle, with failure of the cement at the tip of the stem, may lead to fragmentation of the cement – proximally medially.

Lack of clearance at the anatomical calcar, and hence absence of the stem support proximally posteriorly, is the common finding. Mechanically – lack or loss of the proximal stem support in the presence of good distal fixation is the typical picture. Clinically – active, heavy male after years of excellent function presents with sudden pain which may come on after an apparently normal act like stepping down a step or a sudden turn (Fig. 42.5).

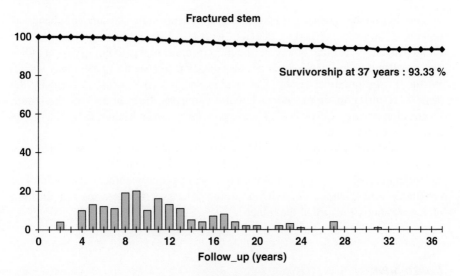

Fig. 42.4 Revision for fractured stem. Incidence and survivorship

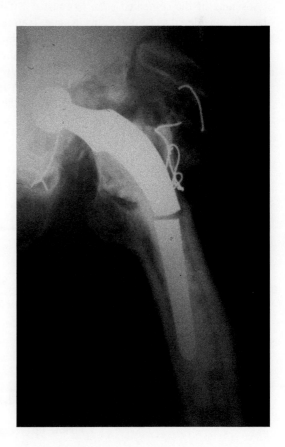

Fig. 42.5 Radiograph
showing stem fracture

This signals the end point of what is fatigue fracture – the mechanism is bending-torsion of the proximal part of the stem with a well fixed distal portion [3]. The initial pain may settle and divert the attention from the real pathology. Urgent radiograph (AP and lateral) is essential because the short free stem fragment may lead to fracture of the proximal femur. The mechanism of stem fracture is basically the same as resulting in slipped upper femoral epiphysis, fracture neck of the femur, localisation of Legg Calve Perthes and avascular necrosis lesions, as well as some cases of osteoarthritis.

Fractured stem after primary LFA is now largely of historical interest. Improved materials (ORTRON: DePuy International, Leeds UK), stem design [4], and surgical technique [5] have eliminated the problem in primary surgery. The effects of proximal strain shielding of the femur present later as a more serious complication of periprosthetic fracture of the femur.

Loose Stem

Loosening of the cemented stem is unusual within the first 4 years and may be largely considered to be due to inadequate fixation or alternatively excessive loading in heavy patients. The "at risk" radiographic appearances have been documented: [6] demarcation of cement at the tip of the stem, fracture cement at the tip of the stem, valgus stem position. Separation of the stem from cement – not significant as a single factor, gains significance when in combination with other signs described. Endosteal cavitation is rarely seen in the first year. Its appearance, at any stage, spells failure and frequent reviews are essential. Stems that are revised for loosening fail between the 5th and 20th year with a survivorship at 37 years follow-up of 74.71 % (Fig. 42.6).

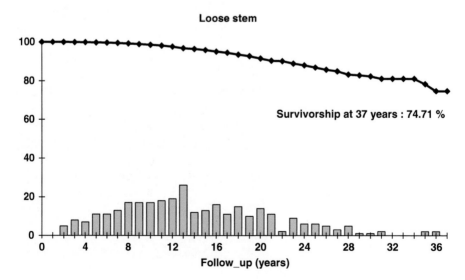

Fig. 42.6 Revision for loose stem. Incidence and survivorship

Normal and unchanged appearance with the stem in neutral, central, position is a good indicator of long-term success. The frequency of review will be dictated by the early radiographic appearance – be this normal or abnormal. But it must be remembered that progression of stem loosening may be very rapid. Within months rather than years bone stock loss may become very extensive. The reason for this is better understood if it is accepted that any change in radiodensity, within the medullary canal, is concealed by the layers of the radiodense cortex. The more radiodense the cortex, the later will the changes be observed on radiographs and more extensive when examined at revision. This explains the discrepancy between radiographic and operative findings and confirms the need for early intervention, for radiographic changes alone.

Increasing incidence of periprosthetic fractures with "cementless" stems may not be merely a reflection of the lack of follow-up but because the stem is loose! (Fig. 42.7)

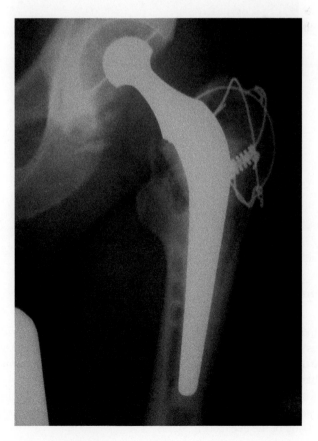

Fig. 42.7 Radiograph of a loose stem

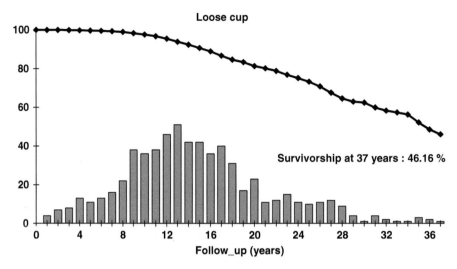

Fig. 42.8 Revision for loose cup. Incidence and survivorship

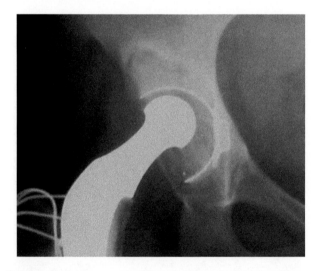

Fig. 42.9 Radiograph of a loose cup

Loose Cup

Wear and loosening of the cemented cup is rare within 4 years of primary surgery and presents numerically as a problem from 8 years onwards (Fig. 42.8). Excluding progressive demarcation, which occurs with infection, early cup loosening or migration is probably the reflection of the surgical technique.

Changes at the bone-implant interface must be looked for in all zones. Although changes superiorly attract attention – changes in the lower cup margin may be a better indication of the events (Fig. 42.9).

The failure occurs at the bone-cement interface. Demarcation of the bone cement, more extensive than the outer one third of the cup [7], on the 1 year radiograph indicates a higher probability of failure with increasing follow-up. Complete demarcation of the bone-cement interface of 2 mm or more is accepted as cup loosening [7]. Migration is defined as change in cup position or orientation as observed on serial radiographs. The incidence of cup loosening and revision is related to the depth of cup penetration. It increases from the fourth year onwards and is an indication of patients activity level. The survivorship at 37 years was 46.16 % (Fig. 42.8).

A high penetration rate of the UHMWPE cup is not compatible with long-term success; long-term successful results show low penetration of the cup [8].

A loose cup is clinically asymptomatic. If progressive loosening and loss of bone stock is to be avoided, then regular follow-up and revisions for radiographic changes alone must be the accepted practice.

Metal Sensitivity

Metal sensitivity has been suggested as a possible cause of failure of total hip replacement. Rooker and colleagues [9] reviewed the literature on the subject and tested 212 patients for sensitivity to nickel, chromium and cobalt, before hip replacement. Fourteen patients showed positive reaction, 62 with history of metal allergy gave a negative patch test, 4 with positive tests had a successful hip replacement with a 2 year follow-up. The authors have also shown that using a metal on plastic prosthesis can sensitise a patient within 6 months after the operation: but concluded that aseptic loosening was not caused by metal sensitivity.

In a study involving 493 patients baseline cutaneous sensitivity to chromium, nickel and cobalt was assessed before and after the use of metallic implants. The prevalence of sensitivity was low: 0.2 %, 1.3 % and 1.8 % to chromium, nickel and cobalt respectively. The range of conversion from negative to positive and from positive to negative was similarly low [10].

Christiansen [11] suggested lymphocyte stimulation index to evaluate an in vitro metal sensitivity in patients with failed total hip prosthesis. Lymphocyte transformation to chromium, cobalt and nickel was measured in 15 patients having revision for loose prostheses and compared with 12 successful controls with a follow-up of at least 2 years.

Positive response (lymphocyte stimulation index of more than three) to at least one of the metals was found in 73 % of the revision group compared with 8 % of controls (p<0.001). A prospective study [12] of allergic contact dermatitis was undertaken in 69 patients undergoing metal on plastic total hip replacement and 54 were available for review after surgery. The authors suggested that cutaneous sensitivity may be the result and not the cause of loosening, and that a metal on plastic combination can be used routinely and that patch testing was no longer required. Pazzaglia and colleagues [13] studied 20 patients with Charnley low-friction arthroplasty with a follow-up of 10–13 years measuring concentration of nickel, chromium and manganese in blood, plasma and urine using atomic absorption spectrophotometry, as well as carrying out skin tests and radiographic assessment

Table 42.1 Details of the seven patients studied

Case number	Gender	Age at LFA (years)	Diagnosis	Metal sensitivity	Sensitivity			Follow-up (years)
					Cr	Co	Ni	
1	F	35	A/S	X			√	30
2 Bilateral LFAs	F	66	OA	XX	√		√	22
3	M	67	OA	X	√			20
4	F	66	OA/ITO	XX	√		√	11
5 Bilateral LFAs	F	64	OA	XX	√		√	8
6	F	59	Sepsis Tb	XX	√		√	23
7	F	32	CDS/OA	X	√	√	√	10

A/S Ankylosing spondylitis, *O/A* Osteoarthritis, *ITO* Intertrochanteric osteotomy, *CDS/OA* Congenital dislocation/dysplasia subluxation with osteoarthritis
X, patch test; XX, history of skin reaction on contact with various items of jewellery

of the arthroplasties. Their conclusion was that "metal – plastic prostheses do not seem to cause sensitisation even after a prolonged period of time" [11]. Histological studies of periprosthetic tissues failed to show any evidence of delayed hypersensitivity [14].

We first came across the problem of a well documented metal (chromium) sensitivity in a patient in 1978. A practical routine was established and we present our experience with the method.

Patients who volunteered a well documented or a strongly suspicious history of cutaneous sensitivity to nickel, chromium or cobalt were given a Charnley stainless steel prosthesis to wear round their neck as a pendant, next to the skin, at all times while awaiting surgery (with time it became more convenient and less cumbersome to wear a smaller "pendant" of a bullet shaped distal fragment of the stem). If any irritation or rash occurred the pendant was to be removed and the result reported.

Seven patients undergoing a Charnley low friction arthroplasty (LFA) were included in the study (Table 42.1). None reported skin sensitivity to the Charnley stem and at a mean follow-up of 18 years and 8 months (8–30 years) there were no failures either clinically or radiologically. At the latest follow-up all patients were pain free and had full or near full range of movements.

One case was of special interest. A female aged 60 developed areas of cellulitis posterior to the incision following bilateral LFAs. This occurred spontaneously and was associated with rigors and an elevated erythrocyte sedimentation rate. It settled with Penicillin but recurred once. The clinical picture was that of streptococcal skin infection – Erysipelas. There were no further problems with normal looking radiographs at 22 years. Unilateral appearance, a clinical picture of infection and response to antibiotics was against metal sensitivity. This condition has been reported recently [15].

Skin sensitivity to various metals, may be volunteered by patients undergoing hip replacement surgery. Our follow-up to 30 years is reassuring: no ill effects have been observed in patients with known metal sensitivity to chromium, cobalt or nickel. For patients who may be worried about this aspect, wearing of a pendant shaped from the off cut of a reject implant, close to the skin is a reasonable reassurance. For obvious reasons we avoided strapping the metal next to the skin.

With the passage of time and increasing experience, the subject of metal sensitivity seems to have been abandoned.

Summary

Dramatic pain relief following the operation is due to the neuropathic nature of the implant. Clinical results do not reflect the mechanical state of the arthroplasty. Follow-up facilities are essential, the frequency of visits will be governed by the documented pattern of radiographic changes and early revision, and not by patients symptoms. Immediate post-operative radiograph is essential; it is a record of the procedure and a baseline for future comparisons.

Progressive loosening, deteriorating function, but above all preservation of bone stock, are the absolute indications for revision.

If follow-up and revision facilities are not offered the question must be: who should bear the continuing burden of clinical, moral, financial and legal responsibility?

> *Everybody operated and everywhere hardly a single surgeon has an opportunity to follow-up his cases, continuity of treatment an essential desideratum was impossible.* **Sir Robert Jones 1915** [16]

Incorrect Identification of the Original Pathology

Hip joint is deep seated and symptoms arising from it have not received detailed attention. The source of symptoms is poorly understood and not sufficiently localised as to be of diagnostic value. Few clinical records carry information beyond the statement: "hip pain". It could be that an obvious limp or the use of a stick for support focuses the attention on the relevant anatomy. Combined with the radiograph already on view, before the history or examination is even carried out, sets the pattern of matching the history of examination to the x-ray image.

Exclusion of spinal pathology as the possible root of symptoms is essential. Local, extra-articular lesions are rare but must be looked for if there is even a slightest doubt.

Inappropriate Patient Selection

There are some individuals that are never satisfied, even with the best service offered in whatever sphere of life. Publicity in the media of single case success may increase the expectations to above the level that can be achieved with surgery. When combined with a small dose of flattery it may divert the surgeon's attention from the main problem. Barring complications, hip replacement offers a clearly defined benefit – **pain relief**. The outcome, both the short and the long-term, depends on the understanding and acceptance of these facts. Patients cannot expect, and the surgeon is not in a position to offer a fulfilment of unrealistic expectations.

References

1. Kaplan EL, Meier P. Nonparametric estimation from incomplete observations. J Am Stat Assoc. 1958;53:457–81.
2. Lettin AF, Ware HS, Morris RW. Survivorship analysis and confidence intervals: an assessment with reference to the Stanmore total knee replacement. J Bone Joint Surg (Br). 1991;73-B:729–31.
3. Wroblewski BM. The mechanism of fracture of the femoral prosthesis in total hip replacement. Int Orthop (SICOT). 1979;3:137–9.
4. Charnley J. Low-friction arthroplasty of the hip. Theory and practice. Berlin: Springer; 1979. p. 125–33.
5. Wroblewski BM, Fleming PA, Hall RM, Siney PD. Stem fixation in the Charnley low friction arthroplasty in young patients using an intramedullary bone block. J Bone Joint Surg (Br). 1998;80-B:273–8.
6. Pacheco V, Shelley P, Wroblewski BM. Mechanical loosening of the stem in Charnley arthroplasties. J Bone Joint Surgery (Br). 1988;70-B:596–9.
7. Hodgkinson JP, Shelley P, Wroblewski BM. The correlation between roentgenographic appearances and operative findings at the bone-cement junction of the socket in the Charnley low-friction arthroplasties. Clin Orthop Relat Res. 1998;228:105–9.
8. Wroblewski BM, Siney PD, Dowson D, Collins SN. Prospective clinical and joint simulator studies of a new total hip arthroplasty using alumina ceramic heads and cross-linked polyethylene cups. J Bone Joint Surg (Br). 1996;78-B:280–5.
9. Rooker GD, Wilkinson JD. Metal sensitivity in patients undergoing hip replacement. A prospective study. J Bone Joint Surg. 1980;62-B:502–5.
10. Swiontkowski MF, Agel J, Schappach J, McNair P, Welch M. Cutaneous metal sensitivity in patients with orthopaedic injuries. J Orthop Trauma. 2001;15:86–9.
11. Christianson KJ. The correlation between prosthesis failure and metal sensitivity as determined by a new immunological technique. J Bone Joint Surg. 1979;61-B:240.
12. Deutman MD, Mulder TJ, Brian R, Nater JP. Metal sensitivity before and after total hip arthroplasty. J Bone Joint Surg. 1977;59A:862–5.
13. Pazzaglia UE, Minoia C, Ceciliani L, Riccardi C. Metal determination in organic fluids of patients with stainless steel hip arthroplasty Acta. Orthop Scand. 1983;54:574–9.
14. Amstutz HC, Grigoris P. Metal on metal bearings in hip arthroplasty. Clin Orthop Relat Res. 1996;3295:511–34.
15. Rodriguez JA, Ranawat CS, Maniar RN, Umlas ME. Functional cellulitis after total hip replacement. J Bone Joint Surg. 1998;80-B:876–8.
16. Watson F. The life of Sir Robert Jones. London: Hodder and Stoughton Ltd; MCMXXXIV. 1915. p. 150.

Chapter 43
Changing Patterns of Patients Presenting for the Operation

Charnley low-frictional torque arthroplasty (LFA) continues to be an evolutionary procedure. Changes in the design materials and surgical technique are introduced as a result of information gathered from long-term follow-up clinical studies, management of complications, findings at revision surgery or examination of explanted components. These changes, modifications and improvements can be seen as being within the control of the individual implementing them, but what about the changes that are independent of that control? Is there a changing pattern of patients presenting for surgery, which may, in the long-term affect the outcome? We reviewed our database in order to establish if there is a discernable changing pattern in patients presenting for surgery.

We have examined the information, collected prospectively, on patients undergoing primary Charnley LFA between November 1962 and December 2014. Included are only those cases where the design, materials and surgical technique conformed with the Charnley concept as practised at that particular stage of the evolution of the operation.

During the 52 year period: 1962–2014, 25,752 primary LFAs, have been carried out. The changing patterns are presented graphically with percentages being part of the whole group.

Gender There is a gradual increase in the number of male patients being accepted for the operation: from the initial 20 % to about 40 % (Fig. 43.1).

Age Since with growing experience younger patients were accepted for the operation, we have taken age 40 years as a dividing level comparing patients aged 40 years or younger with those over 40 years of age. There were 992 patients (3.85 %) aged 40 years or younger at the time of the LFA, the numbers gradually increasing from the early 1970s onwards (Fig. 43.2).

Underlying hip pathology There has been a reduction in the number of patients with rheumatoid arthritis (Fig. 43.3). The most dramatic reduction, from 29 % to below 10 %, occurred in the early 1970s. There have been yearly fluctuations since

© Springer International Publishing Switzerland 2016   331
B.M. Wroblewski et al., *Charnley Low-Frictional Torque Arthroplasty of the Hip: Practice and Results*, DOI 10.1007/978-3-319-21320-0_43

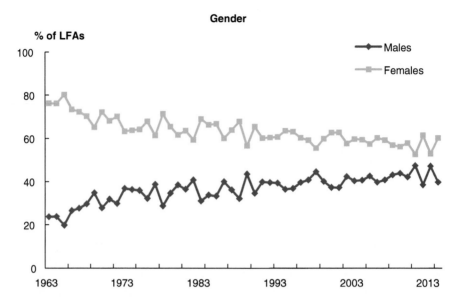

Fig. 43.1 Changing patterns of patients. Graph showing gradual increase in males presenting for hip replacement

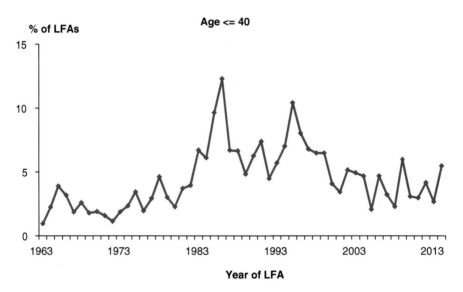

Fig. 43.2 Changing patterns of patients. Younger patients being accepted for hip replacement

but the high levels seen in the 1960s have not been reached. Such a dramatic decline in the early years is unlikely to have been due to the benefits of medical treatments introduced more recently. There has been an increase of patients with osteoarthritis from 60 % to 66 % (Fig. 43.4) and an increase of patients with DDH from 0 % to 10 % (Fig. 43.5).

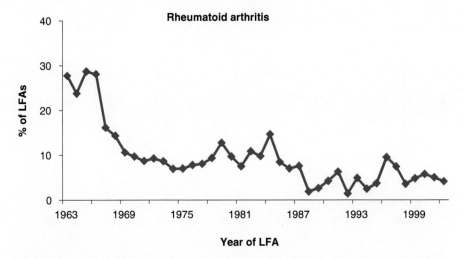

Fig. 43.3 Changing patterns of patients. Reduction in the number of patients with an underlying hip pathology of rheumatoid arthritis

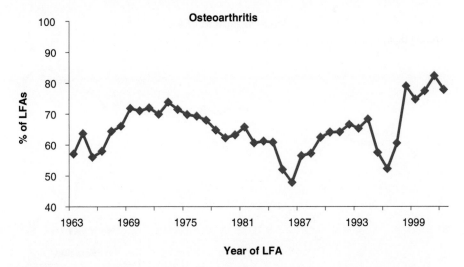

Fig. 43.4 Changing patterns of patients. Increase in the number patients with Osteoarthritis

Previous hip surgery Between the 1970s and early 1980s there has been a gradual increase in the number of patients who have had previous hip surgery. These were primarily patients who had had intertrochanteric osteotomy which had not been successful. Such cases are expected to decline and may, in time, be replaced by the unsuccessful cases of joint preserving procedures.

Weight Patients' weight increased at a mean rate of 0.45 kg/year. The increase for males was from 73 kg to 88 kg and from 59 kg to 72 kg for females (Fig. 43.6). This has implications for the standard of fatigue testing of stemmed femoral components.

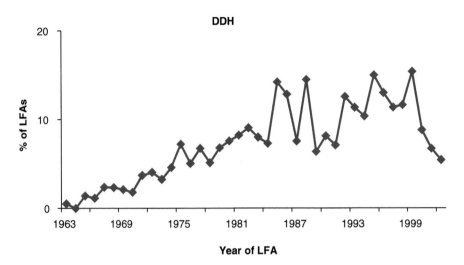

Fig. 43.5 Changing patterns of patients. Increase in the number patients with developmental dysplasia of the hip

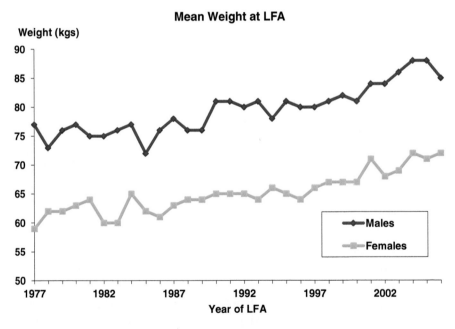

Fig. 43.6 Changing patterns of patients. Increase in patient's weight

The maximum load should be increased from 2.3 to 2.5 kN, while the duration of the test should be increased from 5×10^6 to 10×10^6 cycles to reflect the period at risk for stem fracture [1].

Summary

There is a very definite change in the pattern of patients being accepted for the Charnley LFA. Initially the female patients formed between 70 % and 80 %. The gradual change over the years is clearly demonstrated – with the two genders approaching almost equal ratios.

There is a popular belief that Charnley did not accept young patients for hip replacement. This is not correct. Young patients, with multiple joint involvement, as in rheumatoid arthritis, were accepted as this was the only rational treatment that was available. There has been a dramatic decline in the number of patients with rheumatoid arthritis from 29 % to about 4 % over the 40 year period. This change cannot be explained by the decrease in the number of female patients which has been gradual, or due to more recent advances in the medical treatment: the change is too dramatic and not recent. The change occurred in the 60s/70s and there has not been a corresponding drop more recently. It is likely that patients with rheumatoid arthritis have their hip replacement carried out locally. Would it be too hopeful to suggest that the incidence of rheumatoid arthritis is on the decline?

Confidence in the method, supported by the successful clinical results, extended the indications to younger patients. This is reflected in the increasing number of patients with osteoarthritis secondary to DDH being accepted for surgery. The advent of hip replacement surgery has all but eliminated other forms of treatment for a hip destroyed by arthritis. Intertrochanteric osteotomy as a method of treatment of osteoarthritic hips has been largely abandoned. Few surgeons have an opportunity to find indications, gain practical experience and convey with confidence the benefits of hip fusion.

Our review has shown that there is a changing pattern in the patients presenting for the operation of the Charnley LFA – the number of males under the age of 40, with a diagnosis of osteoarthritis both primary and secondary to DDH increasing, while the number of females, over the age of 40 with rheumatoid arthritis is declining. The patients are getting heavier. It could be argued that the information we present reflects the practice from a Specialist Unit and does not reflect the experience of this type of surgery in a more general set-up. This argument may be correct, but could a non-specialist unit gather sufficient material, with the consistency of all aspects of this type of surgery, and have a long enough follow-up to make a statement of the fact? The changing pattern affecting the outcome demands a review of the design, materials, surgical technique or even patient selection – a mammoth task for a non-specialist unit where elective surgery may have to take second place imposed by emergencies.

The effect of this changing pattern on the long-term results is a subject worth a detailed study. Advances in hip replacement surgery may, initially, be measured by documenting specific aspects in a general population of patients, but will eventually have to be judged by the results imposed by the changing pattern of patients presenting for surgery.

Reference

1. Wroblewski BM, Siney PD, Fleming PA. Increasing patients' body mass. Are the criteria for testing stemmed femoral components in total hip arthroplasty still valid? Proc Inst Mech Eng H. 2007;221(8):959–61.

Chapter 44
Increasing Follow-Up: Changing Age Patterns

The terms "young" patient and "long-term" results are frequently used. Although the age of patients, at surgery, and the length of follow-up are stated, the correlation between the two has not been established. As a result any comparison between published series is largely subjective.

What has not been considered, and has not been documented, is that increasing follow-up must out of necessity, identify ever younger patients that have undergone the operation.

Patients' mean age, both at the primary operation and the follow-up was recorded from November 1962 and December 2014 in 25752 primary LFAs (Tables 44.1 and 44.2, and Fig. 44.1).

The patients mean age at LFA was 64.8 years (range, 13–96). With increasing follow-up the mean age of patients, at the primary LFA and still available for follow-up, decreased by approximately 8 months for each year of follow-up: from 64.8 years (13–96) in the first year to 38.4 years (24–59) at 35 years follow-up when 64 were still available for follow-up.

The mean age of the patients, at the follow-up, increased by approximately 3 months for every year of follow-up: from: 64.8 years (13–96) in the first year to 73.4 years (60–94) at 35 years follow-up.

Survival does favour the young; increasing follow-up identifies increasingly younger patients that have undergone the operation, the underlying hip pathology changes: juvenile idiopathic arthritis (JIA) and secondary arthritis become more prominent [1].

Multiple joint involvement of JIA may not pose a challenge in the way of activity level, but certainly does so with the quality of bone stock for component fixation.

Patients with secondary arthritis will pose technical problems as with developmental hip dysplasia and long-term high activity level with unilateral hip pathology. The challenge to achieve successful results past 40-year follow-up will come from patients age 35 years or younger with secondary and inflammatory hip pathology.

© Springer International Publishing Switzerland 2016
B.M. Wroblewski et al., *Charnley Low-Frictional Torque Arthroplasty of the Hip:
Practice and Results*, DOI 10.1007/978-3-319-21320-0_44

Table 44.1 Mean age and age range at time of LFA

Follow up (years)	Age at LFA (mean)	Range	
		Minimum	Maximum
Operation	64.8	13	96
10	55.9	13	86
20	48.9	14	75
30	43.0	17	63
35	38.4	24	59

Table 44.2 Mean age and age range at time of follow-up

Follow up (years)	Age at follow-up (mean)	Range	
		Minimum	Maximum
Operation	64.8	13	96
10	65.9	23	96
20	68.9	34	95
30	72.9	48	93
35	73.4	60	94

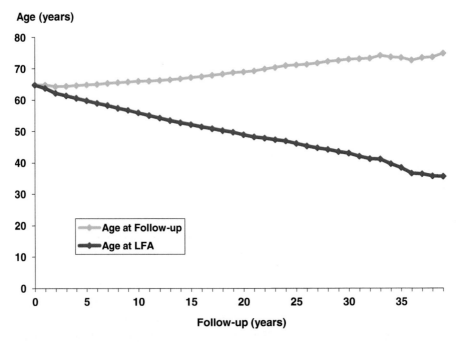

Fig. 44.1 Long-term follow-up identifies younger patients that have undergone a hip replacement

The successful follow-up results to 47 years have been achieved with the original design, materials and the surgical technique [2] and they confirm the Charnley LFA concept. This group of patients offers the most valuable information concerning clinical results [3] radiographic appearances [4] and the study of the explanted materials and components [5, 6].

The long-term results of the Charnley LFA are the results in young patients.

References

1. Wroblewski BM, Purbach B, Siney PD, Fleming PA. Charnley low-friction arthroplasty in teenage patients. The ultimate challenge. J Bone Joint Surg (Br). 2010;92B:486–8.
2. Charnley J. Low friction arthroplasty of the hip in rheumatoid arthritis. Vienna: SICOT; 1963. p. 168–70. Extract of symposium II.
3. Wroblewski BM, Siney PD, Fleming PA. Charnley low-frictional torque arthroplasty: follow-up 30–40 years. J Bone Joint Surg (Br). 2009;91:447–50.
4. Hodgkinson JP, Shelley P, Wroblewski BM. The correlation between the roentgenographic appearance and operative findings at the bone-cement junction of the socket in Charnley low friction arthroplasties. Clin Orthop. 1988;228:105–8.
5. Hall RM, Craig PS, Hardaker C, Siney PD, Wroblewski BM. Measurement of wear in retrieved acetabular sockets. Proc Inst Mech Eng. 1995;209:233–42.
6. Hall RM, Siney PD, Unsworth A, Wroblewski BM. The effect of surface topography of retrieved femoral heads on the wear of UHMWPE sockets. Med Eng Phys. 1997;19(N8):711–9.

Appendix A: John Charnley Research Institute

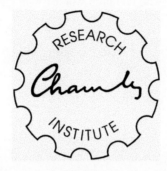

It is essential that the technical skills acquired by members of the staff of a special surgical centre should be handed on continuously so as to keep a body of men capable of handling the difficult secondary operations of the future.

The John Charnley Research Institute was established in 1987 with support from the Peter Kershaw and John Charnley Trusts to continue Charnley's work. Excellent clinical results had created the demand for the Charnley hip replacement, and as a result a number of new issues were identified and addressed.

1. Training of surgeons in the Charnley technique
2. Follow-up facilities with detailed documentation of information including complications and indications for revision
3. Expertise in revision surgery and management of complications
4. Studying the long-term clinical results and explanted materials
5. Advancement of implant materials and designs and operating techniques based on clinical and radiological evidence
6. Dissemination of information through teaching sessions, scientific meetings and publications

Twenty five Clinical Fellows undertook training to further their knowledge and understanding in primary and revision hip replacement and in particular the work of Charnley.

Fifteen of the Fellows were from the UK and Ireland; John Hodgkinson, David Allen, David Beverland, Anthony Browne, Martin Stone, Shiv Gupta, Peter Kay, Videsh Raut, Mike Manning, Anthony Clayson, Eric Gardner, Roger Tillman, Chris Walker, Keith Barnes and Andrew Phillipson.

Four Fellows were from Europe; Blaise Wyssa, Rabih Makarem, Peter Bobak and Bodo Purbach.

Two Fellows were from North and South America, Alberto Dominguez and Major Greg Taylor.

Three Fellows were from Australia, Julian Lane, Scott Crawford and David Mitchell.

© Springer International Publishing Switzerland 2016
B.M. Wroblewski et al., *Charnley Low-Frictional Torque Arthroplasty of the Hip: Practice and Results*, DOI 10.1007/978-3-319-21320-0

The last Fellow Hagime Nagai from Japan completed his fellowship in 2002.

Scott Crawford and Hajime Nagai had followed their respective fathers, Bill Crawford and Jun Nagai, who had both worked with Charnley at Wrightington in the 1960s.

Appendix B: The Biomechanical Laboratory and Workshop

Total hip replacement demands training in mechanical techniques which, though elementary in the practical engineering, are as yet unknown in the training of a surgeon.

One of my aims is to indicate the need for establishing surgical centres to concentrate on the study of the reconstructive surgery of the hip joint.

The Biomechanical Laboratory at Wrightington was opened by Sir Harry Platt in 1961 (Fig. B1). Charnley had persuaded the Manchester Regional Hospital Board's research committee to fund the building of the workshop (Figs. B2 and B3) and it became the focal point for research in gait analysis and biomechanics, wear and materials testing, wound healing and infection. Prototypes for implants and instruments were made and tested on site.

Charnley funded his research at Wrightington with grants from research sponsors and from royalties from the sale of his prostheses manufactured by Chas F Thackray Ltd. He was fortunate to have support in the Biomechanical Laboratory from his dedicated research staff. In the late 1950s, Harry Craven worked with Charnley developing prototype instruments and making the PTFE sockets. It was Craven who in 1962 had tested the new plastic – High molecular weight Polyethylene (HMWPE). In 1966 Geoff Middleton took charge of the laboratory and as the workload increased he was joined by Ken Marsh. In 1973 Frank Brown replaced Geoff Middleton and worked in the laboratory until he retired in 2014. Surgeons were encouraged to spend time in the laboratory working with the technicians to improve their technical skills.

Many thousands of surgeons have visited Wrightington to see first-hand the pioneering work of Charnley (Fig. B4). They have seen first-hand the wear testing equipment (Figs. B5, B6, B7, and B8), the pendulum comparator rig used to demonstrate the principle of low frictional torque (Fig. B9) and the lapping and polishing machine designed to create a perfectly smooth round head on the femoral component (Fig. B10). All these machines had been designed and made in the workshop at Wrightington.

Part of the Laboratory was later converted into a museum in the 1970s showing the history of evolution of the LFA complete with a full size replica of the original clean air enclosure (Greenhouse). It continued to be a place where surgeons and patients could visit and appreciate the pioneering work of Charnley.

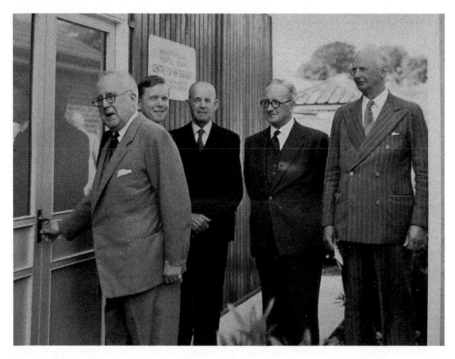

Fig. B1 Photograph of Sir Harry Platt with John Charnley at the opening the Biomechanical Laboratory in 1961

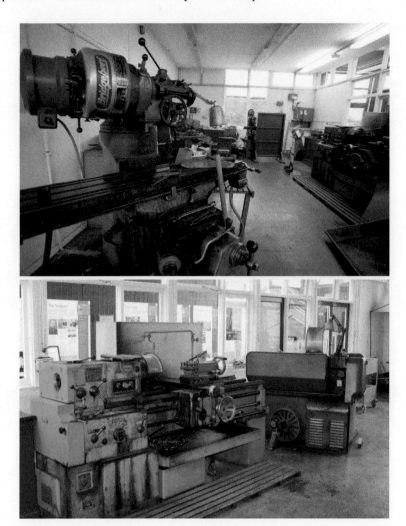

Figs. B2 and B3 The inside of the biomechanical workshop showing some of the machines used to make the implants and instruments

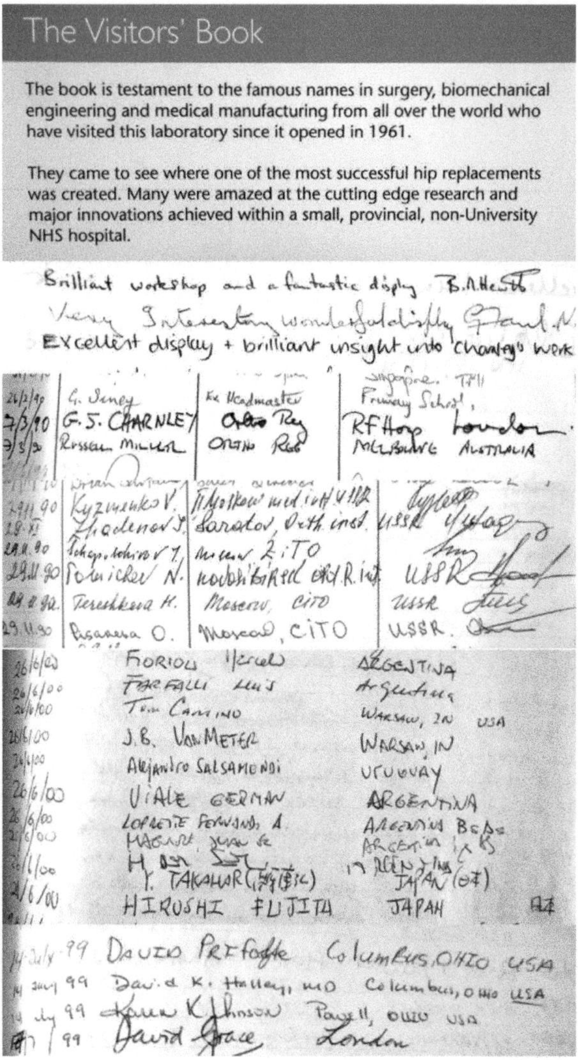
The Visitors' Book
The book is testament to the famous names in surgery, biomechanical engineering and medical manufacturing from all over the world who have visited this laboratory since it opened in 1961.
They came to see where one of the most successful hip replacements was created. Many were amazed at the cutting edge research and major innovations achieved within a small, provincial, non-University NHS hospital.
Brilliant workshop and a fantastic display
Excellent display + brilliant insight into Charnley's work
G. S. CHARNLEY
J.B. VanMETER WARSAW, IN
HIROSHI FUJITA JAPAN
Columbus, Ohio USA
David Grace London

Fig. B4 The Visitors book from the Biomechanical Laboratory, showing some of the names and comments from surgeons and patients

Fig. B5 The first wear
testing machine designed
at Wrighington

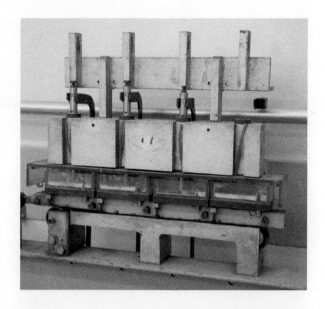

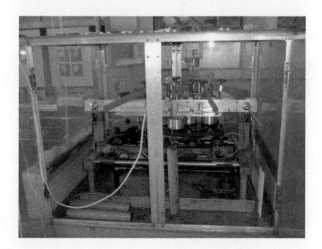

Fig. B6 The pin on plate
wear testing machine

Fig. B7 Close up of the
wear testing machine, the
vertical rods have plastic
tips that moved against the
metal circular discs

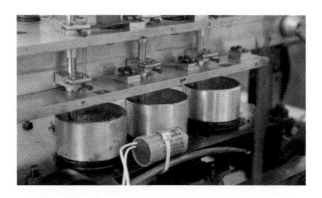

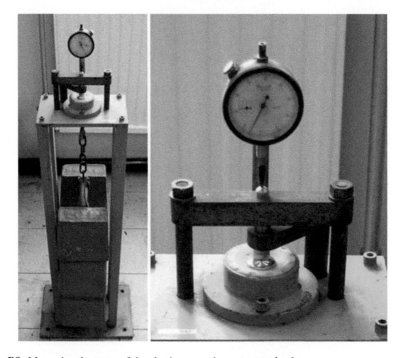

Fig. B8 Measuring the creep of the plastic cup under a constant load

Fig. B9 Pendulum comparator manufactured in the workshop to demonstrate the frictional resistance between various types of femoral heads and acetabular sockets. The pendulums were released simultaneously applying an equal load. The Charnley LFA (small diameter stainless steel femoral head and high density polyethylene socket) kept on swinging when the other side with a larger diameter prosthesis (metal on metal) had ground to a halt

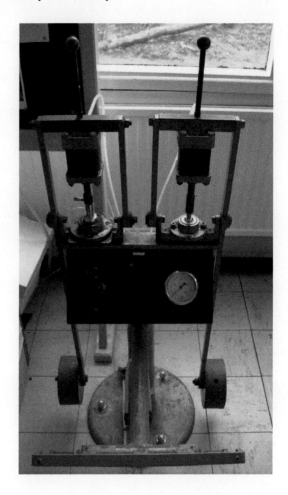

Fig. B10 Lapping and polishing machine designed to create a perfectly smooth round head on the femoral component

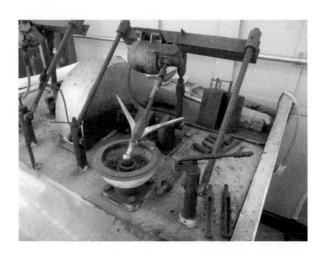

Index

A
Acetabular reaming
    proximal direction, 133–134
    "teardrop" level, 134
    transverse direction, 133–134
Acrylic casts, 259, 260, 264
Acrylic cement
    antibiotic release, 123–125
    bone cements, 19
    cement spacers, 125
    CMW plain *vs.* Gentamicin, 121–122
    ex-vivo study, 123
    femur, 19
Aetiology
    osteoarthritic hips, 52
    primary, unilateral, 52, 53
Angle bore cup, 157–158
Arc of movement, hip joint
    chamfer, 151–152
    head diameter, 150
    labrum and offset, 152
    neck diameter, 150–151
Arthroplasty technique, 49
Aseptic cup loosening, 259, 261

B
Bacteriology, deep infection, 112, 114
Bilateral Charnley press-fit cups, cemented
        stems, 316
Biomechanical Laboratory, 342, 343, 345
Biomechanical workshop
    implants and instruments, 342, 344
    lapping and polishing machine, 349
    pendulum comparator rig, 342, 348
    wear testing machine, 342, 346, 347

Biplaner trochanteric osteotomy
    advantages, 79–80
    disadvantages, 80
    fixation methods and radiographic results,
        80, 83
    Gigli saw, 80–82
Bone cement interphase
    clinical results, 32
    C-stem, 222
    cup demarcation, 239–240
    cup loosening, 241–243
    d'Aubigne and Postel classification, 31
    low-frictional torque, 253
    operative findings, 240
    patients letters to Charnley, 28–29
    post mortem specimens, 27, 30, 32
    radiographic appearances, 31, 33, 240

C
Celestial parallax, 207
Cemented stem and PTFE cup, 10–11
Cement ingress
    acrylic cement, 271, 273, 274
    cup articulating surface, 271
    explanted femoral component, 271–273
Cementless techniques, 245
Charnley acetabular cup
    bore, 227–228
    design evolution, 227
    LPW, 229–230, 232
    ogee flanged cup, 230–232
    PIJ flange, 228, 231
    UHMWPE scalloped cup design
        acetabular reamer, 228, 230
        cup size, 228

© Springer International Publishing Switzerland 2016
B.M. Wroblewski et al., *Charnley Low-Frictional Torque Arthroplasty of the Hip:
Practice and Results*, DOI 10.1007/978-3-319-21320-0

CPI Antony Rowe
Chippenham, UK
2017-01-26 22:37

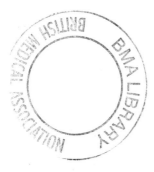